Communication Skills in Pharmacy Practice

A Practical Guide for Students and Practitioners

Third Edition

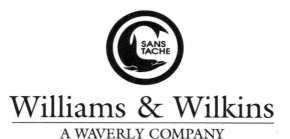

Williams & Wilkins
A WAVERLY COMPANY

BALTIMORE • PHILADELPHIA • LONDON • PARIS • BANGKOK
BUENOS AIRES • HONG KONG • MUNICH • SYDNEY • TOKYO • WROCLAW

Executive Editor: Michael Brown
Development Editor: Fran Klass
Project/Manuscript Editor: Raymond Lukens
Production Manager: Samuel A. Rondinelli

Williams & Wilkens
351 West Camden Street
Baltimore, Maryland 21201-2436 USA

Rose Tree Corporate Center
1400 North Providence Road
Building II, Suite 5025
Media, Pennsylvania 19063-2043 USA

Library of Congress Cataloging-in-Publication Data

Communication skills in pharmacy practice: a practical guide for
students and practitioners / [edited by] William N. Tindall,
Robert S. Beardsley, Carole L. Kimberlin. -- 3rd ed.
    p.   cm.
Includes bibliographical references and index.
ISBN 0-8121-1633-X
    1. Communication in pharmacy. 2. Pharmacist and patient.
I. Tindall, William N. II. Beardsley, Robert S. III. Kimberlin,
Carole L.
    [DNLM: 1. Communication. 2. Pharmacists--[psychology.
3. Professional-Patient Relations. QV 21 C7348 1994]
    RS56.C65   1994
    615'.1'014--dc20   1 ⊘𝒟 l ʦⲟ S ʰ l ✗
    DNLM/DLC
    for Library of Congress   93-6170
    CIP

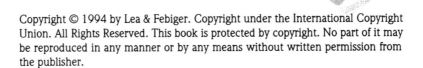

Printed in the United States of America.

Print number: 5 4 3

To
Sylvia, Christine and Laura;
Kathy, Kyle;
and Philip
  for
Communicating the Lessons of Love

Preface

We live in times when patients display voracious appetites for information about their medications. This phenomenon is occurring at the same time that a growing body of professional and lay literature is arguing for, and substantiating the need for, cost-effective pharmacist-based services that include face-to-face counseling. Today, pharmacists are focusing on providing value-added, patient-centered services commonly referred to as pharmaceutical care. The need for pharmaceutical care is further supported by research stating that more than half of the 1.7 billion prescriptions dispensed each year are taken incorrectly. Further support for pharmacists' value-added professional services consists of statements from such notables as former Surgeon General Everett C. Koop, M.D., who says, "There is no substitute for a pharmacist's dialogue ... and the pharmacist should be compensated for services above the dispensing of a product."

Mandates contained in the new Omnibus Budget Reconciliation Act of 1990 (OBRA '90) require pharmacists to offer patient counseling to Medicaid patients. In addition, nearly all 50 states have redefined their statutory definition of "dispensing" to include a patient-counseling component. These laws now empower pharmacists to become more active in assuring that patients understand their medication and can reach the desired outcome of their medication regimen. In fact, the Joint Commission of Pharmacy Practitioners (JCPP) has publicly stated that the mission of pharmacy practitioners "is to help people get the best use of their medicine."

We believe that most pharmacists have always known what information should be taught to patients. This book's mission is to help pharmacists become better teachers by becoming better communicators. This in turn will help pharmacists meet their responsibilities as helping professionals. Improving ones interpersonal communication skills is based upon understanding and assimilating certain processes such as developing an empathic, caring attitude, becoming an effective listener, receiving and providing appropriate feedback, and other skills discussed in this book.

This book breaks interpersonal communications down into its components and stresses its practical application to pharmacy. It begins with a prologue that centers on the importance of communication in meeting a pharmacist's responsibilities by taking the patient's viewpoint. In fact, this "viewpoint of the patient" has become the center of a great paradigm shift in pharmacy, i.e., away from a product in a delivery system and toward a service meeting the needs of a patient. Part I focuses on the interpersonal communication model, the importance of perceptions, barriers that hinder communication, and the role of nonverbal distractions. Part II explains practical life skills that facilitate communication: listening, empathic responding, and assertiveness. Empathic responding or active listening is included because too often false assumptions are made about listening. The assertiveness chapter is helpful in maintaining self-respect and the respect of others in critical situations.

The last third of the book brings specific attention to strategies for improving patient understanding of their medication as the key element in assuring compliant behavior. Interviewing techniques, communication needs of special patients, and ethical patient care are offered as tools to sharpen the skills presented in the first six chapters.

This third edition of *Communication Skills in Pharmacy Practice* was created because of positive support from students, faculty, and practitioners. There are over 60 pharmacy schools both in the USA and abroad that have adopted this book as a teaching text. Feedback from those users and other colleagues has been used to craft revisions for this edition; thus, we hope this new edition's principles, practices, and procedures continue as a worthwhile contribution to better health among those who use America's most trusted professional — their pharmacist.

Alexandria, Virginia	William N. Tindall
Baltimore, Maryland	Robert S. Beardsley
Gainesville, Florida	Carole L. Kimberlin

Contents

PROLOGUE

Communication in the Context of Patient Care

Pharmacists' Responsibility in Patient Care

Importance of Communication in Meeting Patient Care Responsibilities

Understanding Medication Use from the Patient Perspective

Pharmacists are accepting increased responsibility in assuring that patients reach desired outcomes with their drug treatment. This changing role requires pharmacists to switch from a "medication-centered" or "task-centered" practice to "patient-centered" care. Patient-centered care depends on the pharmacist's ability to develop trusting relationships with patients, to engage in an open exchange of information, to involve patients in the decision-making process regarding treatment, and to reach therapeutic goals that are endorsed by patients as well as by health care providers. Effective communication is central to meeting these patient-care responsibilities in the practice of pharmacy.

PHARMACISTS' RESPONSIBILITY IN PATIENT CARE

The cost to society associated with medication-related morbidity and mortality is of growing concern (Hepler & Strand, 1990; Manasse, 1989). The potential of pharmacists to play a pivotal role in reducing the incidence of drug-related illness is likewise receiving increased attention. Hepler and Strand (1990) have made a compelling case for the societal need for pharmaceutical care, which they define as "the responsible provision of drug therapy for the purpose of achieving definite outcomes that improve a patient's quality of life." Mission statements of professional pharmacy associations have been changed in recent years to reflect the increased responsibility pharmacists are being asked to assume for the appropriate use of drugs in society. Such an expanded role for pharmacists is also mandated under provisions of the Omnibus Budget Reconciliation Act of 1990 (OBRA '90), which went into effect in January 1993.

Under provisions of the OBRA legislation, pharmacists are required to obtain information from Medicaid patients or their care givers as well as to provide information to patients for the purpose of preventing or identifying and resolving potential medication-related problems. Pharmacists must maintain patient profiles that contain patient demographic information, a comprehensive list of medications being taken, allergies, adverse drug reactions, disease states, and pharmacist comments relevant to an individual patient's drug therapy. This database can allow pharmacists to fulfill the OBRA requirement of prospective drug-use review, which involves examination of a patient's records prior to dispensing a medication in order to identify and resolve any potential problems that may be apparent. These problems could include over-utilization, under-utilization, therapeutic duplication, drug-drug interactions, incorrect drug dosage, drug-allergy problems, incorrect duration of drug treatment, clinical abuse or misuse, and drug-disease contraindications. In addition, pharmacists are required to offer to engage in a discussion of a patient's therapy whenever a medication is dispensed. Under this provision, a pharmacist must offer to counsel patients on their medications (both new and refill) in order to prevent or identify/resolve problems with medication use.

The "patient-centered" role envisioned by pharmacy mission statements and OBRA '90 provisions would afford pharmacists a value to society far beyond that provided by their current "drug-centered" role. In fact, neither drug products nor dispensing tasks, per se, are essential to a patient-centered mission — these are simply *means* of achieving specified goals in individual patients. The goals are those *outcomes* of therapy that improve a patient's health and quality of life.

However, while the mission statements of professional organizations can help guide practice, they must be translated into patient-care activities that pharmacists provide to each of their patients. The interpersonal relationships professionals develop with patients require effective communication skills and are necessary in meeting a professional mission for pharmacy.

IMPORTANCE OF COMMUNICATION IN MEETING PATIENT CARE RESPONSIBILITIES

The communication process between health professionals and patients serves two primary functions:

1. It establishes the ongoing relationship between the provider and the patient; and

2. It provides the exchange of information necessary to assess a patient's health condition, implement treatment of medical problems, and evaluate the effects of treatment on a patient's quality of life.

Establishing a trusting relationship with a patient is not simply something that is "nice to do" (but essentially peripheral to the "real" purpose of a patient-pharmacist encounter). The quality of the patient-provider relationship is crucial. All professional activities between a pharmacist and a patient take place in the context of the relationship they establish. An effective relationship forms the base which allows a pharmacist to meet professional responsibilities in patient care.

The ultimate purpose of the professional-patient relationship and of the activities engaged in must constantly be kept in mind. The essential goal is to be able to achieve mutually understood and agreed-upon health outcomes that improve a patient's quality of life. Pharmacist activities must, therefore, be thought of in terms of patient outcomes they help to reach. We must begin to redefine what we do, with the focus being on patient need. Our goal, for example, is changed from providing patients with drug information to that of assuring that patients understand their treatment in order to take medications safely and appropriately. Our goal is not to get patients to do as they are told (i.e., comply), but to help them reach intended treatment outcomes. Providing information or trying to improve compliance must each be seen as a means to reaching a desired outcome rather than being an end in itself. Even communication with a patient is not an end in itself. Conversation between patient and health professional has a different purpose than conversation between friends. Patient-professional communication is a means to an end — that of establishing a therapeutic relationship in order to effectively provide health care services that the patient needs. It is the patient's well-being that is paramount. In addition, professionals, because of their unique knowledge and special societal responsibilities, must bear the greater burden in assuring effective communication in patient-professional encounters.

UNDERSTANDING MEDICATION USE FROM THE PATIENT PERSPECTIVE

Models of the prescribing process that are "practitioner centered" have primarily focused on decisions made and actions taken by physicians and other health care providers. The patient is "acted upon" rather than portrayed as an active participant who makes ongoing decisions affecting the outcomes of treatment. The patient in a "professional-centered" model is presented as the object of professional ministrations and as the cooperative (or recalcitrant) enforcer of professional dictates.

One of our professional conceits seems to be the belief that writing the prescription and dispensing the drug are the key acts in the medication use process. However, in most cases it is the patient or the patient's care giver who must return home and carry out the prescribed treatment. The degree of autonomy that is possible with medication therapy in noninstitutionalized patients makes it likely, in fact, that patients will make decisions and assert control over treatment in various ways. Many patients make autonomous decisions to alter treatment regimens — decisions that may be made without consultation or communication with health care providers (Conrad, 1985; Donovan & Blake, 1992; Trostle, 1988). Ignorance of patient-initiated decisions regarding medication use, in turn, makes it difficult, if not impossible, for health care professionals to accurately evaluate the effects of drug treatment.

While providers no doubt view such patient behavior as misadvised, it would probably be more helpful for them to acknowledge the fact that patients do exercise ultimate control over drug treatment. Rather than trying to stifle patient autonomy, it may be more productive for health professionals to strengthen the therapeutic alliance with patients by increasing the level of patient participation and control in decisions that are made about treatment.

A patient-centered model of the medication-use process (see Figure A) focuses on the patient role in the process ("patient" is used to refer to either the patient or the patient's care giver). The medication-use process for noninstitutionalized patients begins when the patient perceives a health care need or health-related problem. This is experienced as a deviation from what is "normal" for the individual. It may be the experience of "symptoms" or other sort of life-style interruption that challenges or threatens the patient's sense of well-being. The patient then interprets the perceived problem. This interpretation is influenced by a host of psychological and social factors unique to the individual. These include the individual's previous experience with the formal health

Prologue

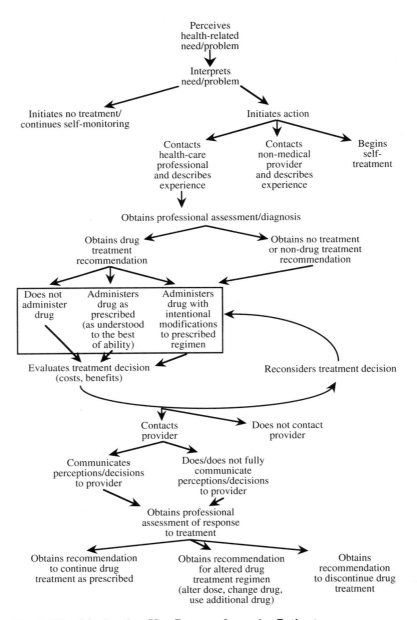

Fig. A. The Medication-Use Process from the Patient Perspective

care system; family influences; cultural differences in the conceptualization of "health" and "illness"; knowledge of the problem (individuals vary greatly on the level of medical and biological knowledge); health beliefs that are more common sense or folk beliefs and may or may not coincide with accepted medical "truths"; psychological characteristics; personal values, motives, and goals; and so on. In addition, the patient's interpretation may be influenced by outside forces, such as family members who offer their own interpretations and advice.

The patient at this point may take no action to treat, either because the problem is seen as minor or transitory or because the patient lacks the means to initiate treatment. If the patient takes action, the action can include initiation of self-treatment, initiation of contact with a non-medical provider (such as a faith healer), and/or contact with a health care provider. (In describing this model, we will only follow the actions regarding medication use as they apply within the formal health care system. A similar process of evaluation and reconsideration regarding treatment would also apply for self-initiated treatment or treatment advised by nonmedical providers.) If the patient takes action that involves contact with a health care professional, whether it be a physician, pharmacist, or other health care practitioner, he must describe his "symptom" experience, and to some extent his interpretation of that experience. In many ways, it is at this point that control gets transferred from the patient to the professional, for it is the professional who can legitimize the experience by giving it a name (diagnosis). Such an act, however, transforms the experience from that with patient meaning into that with practitioner meaning (which may or may not be shared by the patient). The quality of the professional assessment depends, in part, on the thoroughness of the patient report, the skill of the practitioner in eliciting relevant information, and the receptivity of the professional to "hear" information from the patient that is potentially important. The practitioner's skill in communicating information about the diagnosis may alter or refine the patient's conceptualization of his illness experience, making patient understanding more congruent with that of the practitioner.

Once the health care provider reaches a professional assessment or diagnosis of the patient's problem based on patient report, patient examination, and other data, he makes a recommendation to the patient. If the recommendation is to initiate drug treatment, patients may or may not carry out the recommendation for a variety of reasons, including economic constraints, a lack of understanding of the purpose of the recommendation, or failure to "buy into" the treatment plan. Some of these patient decisions may, in fact, reflect failure in the communication process between provider and patient.

When patients do accept the recommendation to initiate drug treatment, obtain the medication, and attempt to follow the regimen as prescribed, they can do so only to the best of their ability as they understand the drugs are intended to be taken. For many patients, medication taking includes misunderstanding of what is recommended or unintended deviations from the prescribed treatment regimen (e.g., doses are forgotten). Alternatively, patients may administer the drug but with intentional modifications of the regimen. In both unintentional and intentional modifications of the prescribed treatment, the patient's actions may be influenced by how well providers succeeded in establishing a mutually understood and agreed-upon treatment plan. Regardless of the medication-taking practices that patients establish, they evaluate the consequences of the treatment in terms of perceived benefits and perceived costs or barriers. This evaluation results in patients continuing with the drug treatment practices essentially as they have been established, patients altering their drug treatment regimens, or patients stopping drug treatment. In any case, patients are continuously estimating what they perceive the effects of their actions to be and adjusting their behavior accordingly. It is inevitable that as patients begin drug treatment, they will "monitor" their own response — they will decide whether or not they feel differently; they will look for signs that the treatment is effective or, alternately, indications that there may be a problem with the drug. The problem is not that patients monitor their response to medications — it is inevitable and desirable that they do so. The problem is that patients often lack information on what to expect from treatment — information that will give them valid feedback on their response to the medication. Lacking this information, they apply their own "common sense" criteria.

Patients may interrupt the treatment process by failing to contact providers when follow-up is expected, which may involve discontinuing participation in the formal health care system for a period of time or contacting a new provider and beginning the whole process again. Other patients may not contact providers because no follow-up was expected and the patient perceives no additional need for provider services. Of the patients who do contact the provider, some will communicate their perceptions, problems, and decisions regarding treatment. Others may contact providers and *not* convey this information (or not convey all pertinent aspects). This follow-up contact occurs during revisits with a physician or refills of prescriptions from pharmacists. The nature of the relationship with the provider; the degree to which the patient feels "safe" in confiding difficulties or concerns; the skill of the provider in eliciting patient perceptions; the extent to which a sense of "partnership" has been established regarding treatment decisions — all influence the patient decision to contact providers and the degree to which medication-taking practices are reported and perceptions shared. Regardless of how completely patients report their experience with therapy when they recontact providers, the provider will make a professional assessment of patient response to treatment based on what the patient does report and/or lab values and other physiological measures. This assessment will lead to recommendations to continue drug treatment as previously recommended, to alter drug treatment (i.e., to change dose, change drug, add drug), or to discontinue drug treatment. This leads once again to patients administering the drug therapy as they understand it and to the best of their ability, altering the treatment, or choosing to not administer the drug. At any point in the process, the patient's evaluation of his condition or treatment may lead back to the beginning (Fig. A) where an altered perception of a health-related need or problem is formed.

Analysis of the medication-use process highlights several things. First, the decision to initiate drug treatment is actually a small part of the process. Secondly, patients and professionals may be carrying out parallel decision making with only sporadic communication about these processes. Furthermore, the communication that does exist may be incomplete and ineffective. Yet both patient and provider continue making decisions and evaluating outcomes regardless of the quality of their understanding of each other's actions and decisions. One of the goals of the communication process should be to make the understanding of the patient and provider regarding the disease, illness experience, and treatment objective as congruent as possible.

It is obvious that there are numerous points in the process where the quality of the patient-professional relationship and the thoroughness of the information exchange affect the decisions of both patients and health professionals. It is at these points that the communication skills of the professional are critical and can have the most effect on the outcomes of treatment.

SUMMARY

In establishing effective relationships with patients, the pharmacist's responsibility to help patients achieve desired health outcomes must be kept in mind. The patient is the focus of the medication-use process. The communication skills of pharmacists can facilitate the formation of trusting relationships with patients as well as establish an open exchange of information and foster a sense of "partnership" between patients and providers. An effective communication process can optimize the chance that patients will make informed decisions, use medications appropriately, and, ultimately, meet therapeutic goals.

REFERENCES

Conrad, P: The meaning of medications: Another look at compliance. Social Science and Medicine, *20*:29-37, 1985.

Donovan JL, & Blake DR: Patient non-compliance: Deviance or reasoned decision-making? Social Science and Medicine, *34*:507-513, 1992.

Hepler CD, & Strand LM: Opportunities and responsibilities in pharmaceutical care. American Journal of Hospital Pharmacy, *47*:533-543, 1990.

Manasse HR: Medication use in an imperfect world: Drug misadventuring as an issue of public policy, part 1. American Journal of Hospital Pharmacy, *46*:929-944, 1989.

Trostle JA: Medical compliance as an ideology. Social Science and Medicine, *27*:1299-1308, 1988.

PART 1

What Is Communication?

CHAPTER *1*

Principles and Elements of Interpersonal Communication

Setting the Stage

Components of the Interpersonal Communication Model

Responsibility of Pharmacists in the Communication Model

In Search of the Meaning of the Message

Words and Their Context

Congruence Between Verbal and Nonverbal Messages

Preventing Misunderstanding

Using Feedback to Check the Meaning of the Message

Toward the Improvement of Communication

OVERVIEW

This chapter describes the process of interpersonal communication as it relates to pharmacy practice. Interpersonal communication is a common but complex practice that is essential in dealing with patients and other health care providers. This chapter also prepares the reader for subsequent chapters, which describe ways of improving interpersonal relations and communication.

SETTING THE STAGE

In our personal and professional lives, we all have to interact with other individuals. Some of these situations are successful; others are not. Consider the following situation: you are a pharmacist working alone in a community pharmacy. George Raymond, a 59-year-old man with moderate hypertension, enters the pharmacy smoking a cigar. You know George because you attend the same church. He is a high school principal, has a wife who works, and has four kids. He has been told to quit smoking and go on a diet, but he has a long history of noncompliance with such requests. He is here to pick up a new prescription: an antibiotic for a urinary tract infection. Although he knows you personally, he is somewhat hesitant as he approaches the prescription area. He looks down at the ground and mumbles, "The doctor called in a new prescription for me, and can I also have a refill of my heart medication?"

In most communication encounters we typically do not have the opportunity to stop and analyze the situation. To improve our communication skills we need some ability to assess a particular situation quickly. Take, for example, the situation just presented. On a piece of paper briefly describe what Mr. Raymond might be thinking or feeling. What clues do you have? Write down what you might say to him. Set the paper aside and read on. Once you have finished the chapter, come back to your notes and rewrite your response based on any insights that resulted from your reading.

COMPONENTS OF THE INTERPERSONAL COMMUNICATION MODEL

Communication in general encompasses a broad spectrum of media; for example, mass communication (TV, radio), small group communication (committee meetings, discussion groups), and large group communication (lectures, speeches). This book focuses on one-to-one, interpersonal communication that occurs in pharmacy practice, such as was observed in the situation with George Raymond. In this section, the interpersonal communication process, or the interaction between two individuals, will be described in detail. This specific form of communication (interpersonal communication) is best described as a process in which messages are generated and transmitted by one person and subsequently received and translated by another. A practical model of this process, as shown in Figure 1-1, combines five important elements: sender, message, receiver, feedback, and barriers.

The Sender. In the interpersonal communication process, the sender transmits a message to another person. In the example given, the initial sender of a message was Mr. Raymond.

The Message. In interpersonal communication, the message is the element that is transmitted from one person to another.

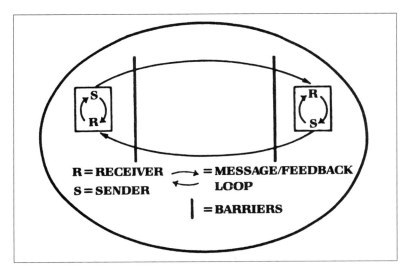

Fig. 1–1. The interpersonal communication model.

Messages can be thoughts, ideas, emotions, information, or other factors, and can be transmitted both verbally (talking) and nonverbally (using facial expressions, hand gestures, etc.). For example, Mr. Raymond's verbal message was that he wanted his new prescription and that he would like to have his prescription for heart medication refilled. He was also communicating nonverbal messages. Did you recognize any of these nonverbal messages? By looking down at the ground and mumbling rather than speaking clearly he might have been expressing embarrassment, shyness, or hesitancy to talk with you. He might have been feeling embarrassed, because he had not been taking his heart pills as he should. As will be discussed later in greater detail in Chapter 2, the nonverbal component of communication is important, because research has found that in some situations 55% or more of a message is transmitted through its nonverbal component.

In most situations, senders formulate or encode messages *before* transmitting them. However, in some cases, messages are transmitted spontaneously without the sender thinking about it, such as a glaring stare or a burst of laughter. In the above situation, Mr. Raymond may not have been aware that he was transmitting nonverbal messages to you.

The Receiver. The receiver (you, the pharmacist in the above example) receives the message from the sender (Mr. Raymond). As the receiver, you "decoded" the message and assigned a particular meaning to it, which may or may not have been the same meaning intended by Mr. Raymond. In translating the message, you considered both the nonverbal and verbal components of the message.

Feedback. Feedback is the process of the initial receiver's communicating back to the initial sender her understanding of the sender's message. By using verbal and nonverbal communication the receiver feeds back information to the sender about how the message was translated. In the feedback loop, the initial receiver becomes the sender of feedback and the initial sender becomes the receiver of feedback, as noted in the model. In the interpersonal communication process, individuals are thus constantly moving back and forth between the roles of sender and receiver. In the above example, you were first a receiver of information, but when you returned feedback to Mr. Raymond you became a sender.

Feedback can be simple, such as merely nodding your head, or more complex, such as repeating a set of complicated instructions. In the above example, feedback would be your response to Mr. Raymond. What did you indicate would be your response to Mr. Raymond? You could have said, "I'm sorry, George, I'm not sure what you are asking. Which medication do you need?" or "How are you feeling, George? You seem a bit down." Feedback allows communication to be a two-way process rather than a one-way monologue. During the communication process, most of us tend to focus on the message and frequently miss the feedback component. We either fail to provide appropriate feedback to the sender when we are the receiver of a message, or we fail to recognize feedback or to ask for feedback when we are the sender of the message. Consequently, we may think that a communication interaction was more effective than it really was. As discussed in Chapter 4, feedback can be strengthened by being sensitive to others and is best done when a person understands the situation in which a message is generated.

Barriers. Interpersonal communication is usually affected by a number of interferences or barriers. These barriers affect the accuracy of the communication exchange. For example, if there was a loud noise in your pharmacy while you were talking to Mr. Raymond, it would be even more difficult to understand what he was trying to communicate. Other physical barriers to your interaction with Mr. Raymond might include a safety glass partition between Mr. Raymond and you, telephones ringing in the background, or Mr. Raymond's defective hearing aid. Additional factors serving as barriers to communication are discussed in Chapter 3.

RESPONSIBILITY OF PHARMACISTS IN THE COMMUNICATION MODEL

A few comments should be made regarding the pharmacist's responsibility in the role of a sender and receiver of messages. As a sender, you are responsible for assuring that the message is transmitted in the clearest form, in terminology understood by the other person, and in an environment conducive to clear transmission. To check if the message was received as intended, you should ask for feedback from the receiver and should clarify any misunderstandings. Thus, your obligation as the sender of a message is not complete until you have determined that the other person has understood it correctly.

As a receiver, you have the responsibility of listening to what is transmitted by the sender. To assure accurate communication, you should provide feedback to the sender by describing what you understood the message to be. We may at times rely on our assumptions that we are understanding each other and thus feel that feedback is not necessary. However, research has found that without appropriate feedback, misunderstandings occur. Of concern is that, as pharmacists dealing with patients, physicians, and other health care providers, can we afford these misunderstandings? Might these misunderstandings result in harm to the patient? To become more effective, efficient, and accurate communicators, we must strive to include feedback in our interactions with others.

In both the role of receiver and sender, you should also be aware of the interference or barriers that exist and attempt to minimize them. Subsequent chapters will illustrate ways to improve your skills as a receiver and a sender of messages and reveal ways to minimize communication barriers.

IN SEARCH OF THE MEANING OF THE MESSAGE

The interpersonal communication model shows how messages originate from a sender and are received by a receiver. The sender delivers the message, and the receiver assigns a meaning to that message. The critical component in this process is that the receiver assign the same meanings to the verbal and nonverbal messages as intended by the sender. In other words, the receiver may or may not interpret the message's meaning in the same way as the sender intended. In the encounter with Mr. Raymond he may not have been embarrassed or hesitant to talk with you at all. Possibly he was looking down at his new tie that he just spilled coffee on. He may have been upset at himself and was concentrating on his predicament rather than on communicating clearly with you. Thus, the message that you received was not the one Mr. Raymond intended.

Words and Their Context

This section discusses how meanings of messages are derived in the interpersonal communication process. In general, individuals assign meaning to verbal and nonverbal messages based on their past experiences and previous definitions of these verbal and nonverbal elements. If two persons do not share the same definition or past experiences, misunderstanding may occur. The most common example of this is evident in different languages and dialects of the world. Different words mean certain things to different people based on the definitions learned. For example, "football" to an American means a sport using an oval ball, but "football" to a European means a sport using a round ball (soccer). An example of this misunderstanding occurs in health care when we speak in medical terminology that may have different (or possibly no) meanings to our patients. The following example illustrates this potential misunderstanding.

In the beginning exercise, let us assume that you wish to inform Mr. Raymond that his urinary tract antibiotic will be more effective if taken with sufficient fluid to guarantee adequate urinary output. You relate that intent in the following words, "This medication should be taken with plenty of fluids." The message is received and decoded into words and symbols in the mind of Mr. Raymond. These words or symbols may or may not have any particular meaning to him; perhaps he does not even know what "fluids" refers to; perhaps he is uncertain if you consider milk to be a fluid; or perhaps he associates the word "plenty" with a small glass of orange juice at breakfast rather than the amount you had in mind. Thus, the meaning of your important message may or may not have been received accurately by Mr. Raymond. It is the assignment of meaning to those words by Mr. Raymond that is important.

The following actual situation is another illustration of this point.

An elderly patient who was taking several medications complained to her pharmacist that she was having trouble taking her potassium. The pharmacist asked, "What seems to be the problem? Are you taking it as instructed?"

The patient replied, "Yes, that's no problem. I take it just like it says on the label: 'Take one tablet each morning in water.' But I prefer to take my bath at night, not in the morning."

Apparently, the patient translated the phrase "in water" to mean that she had to take it when she was physically in water or in her bath. She assigned meaning to those words based on her past experiences of what "in water" referred to. Obviously, her definition of that phrase was not the same as intended by the pharmacist.

Another important factor is that people assign meanings based on the context that they perceive the sender is using. Many times patients will understand the words that we are using but place them in a different context and thus assign a different meaning to our message than the one intended. The following actual situation illustrates this point:

A nine-month-old baby had to be admitted to the hospital with a severe infection because his mother misunderstood the labeled instructions for an antibiotic: "Take one-half teaspoonful three times a day for infection until all gone." The mother continued the drug for about three days until the baby appeared to be getting better. The mother then stopped giving the antibiotic; a superinfection developed and the baby was hospitalized.

In this example, the mother interpreted the directions to mean "give the medication until the infection is all gone." The physician and pharmacist intended to communicate that the medication should be continued until the entire contents of the bottle (10 days' supply) were used up. She understood the words correctly, but she put them into a different context and thus derived a different meaning from the one intended by the pharmacist.

Congruence Between Verbal and Nonverbal Messages

The meaning of the message may be somewhat unclear if the receiver senses an incongruence between the verbal and nonverbal messages. That is, the meaning of a verbal message is not consistent with the meaning of a nonverbal message. The following situations reveal potential incongruent messages:

1. A beet-red-faced patron comes into the pharmacy, raises a fist, and loudly proclaims, "I'm not angry, I'm just here to ask about a prescription error."

2. A disappointed pharmacist has tried for hours to convince a physician to change an obvious error in a patient's medication. When asked how he is feeling, he meekly replies, "Oh, I'm just fine."

3. A patient hands a pharmacist a prescription for a tranquilizer, then bursts into tears. The pharmacist asks if anything is the matter, and the patient responds, "No, I'm okay, it's nothing at all."

In the above examples, it is obvious that the verbal messages did not match the nonverbal messages, and the receiver may be confused about the true message intended by the sender. To avoid this incongruence, as a sender, you must be aware of the nonverbal messages that are sent as well as the verbal messages; as a receiver, you should point out to the sender that you are receiving two different messages.

In summary, people base their interpretation of verbal and nonverbal messages on a variety of factors, including their definition of words and symbols and their perception of the words, symbols, and nonverbal elements used by the sender. It is not what is said, but what the receiver perceives was said. The following section addresses how to prevent possible misunderstandings.

Preventing Misunderstanding

In the previously cited situation involving the baby's antibiotic prescription, the label read, "Take one-half teaspoonful three times a day for infection until all gone." Unfortunately, the mother interpreted the message incorrectly. In this situation, the meaning could be clarified relatively easily by putting the words in a different context by rearranging the position of the last two prepositional phrases (…three times a day until all gone for infection). However, minimizing misunderstandings is many times more difficult in other situations.

We often assume that the receiver will interpret our message accurately. We fail to realize that different people may assign different meanings to words or phrases that we use. We are generally unaware of this fact. To improve the communication process, we must remember that people assign meanings to messages based on their background, values, and experiences. If other persons have different backgrounds, values, and experiences, then they may assign a different meaning to our intended message. Many of our problems in communication occur because we forget that individual experiences are never identical. In actual practice, we have enough common experiences with people we deal with on a daily basis that we can understand each other pretty well. Typically, we can anticipate how patients are feeling and their level of general understanding of what drugs are used for. It is when we have limited common experiences or do not share the same meaning of certain words and symbols that communication breaks down. Thus, a person placed on a medication for the first time or a person of a different gender, age, or race may have different experiences than we do.

A key to preventing misunderstanding is anticipating how other persons may translate your message. It may be helpful to determine their experience with drugs in general and with a particular drug specifically. If they have had positive experiences previously, then their perception of drugs may be different than if they have had bad experiences. If they have negative feelings about drugs, then they may be reluctant to discuss the medication or even take it. Some of the skills discussed in the chapter on empathic listening may be helpful in anticipating how others may assign meaning to your message. In many communication interactions, the more you know about other persons and the more you are able to understand them, the easier it will be to anticipate how they may interpret the meaning of the message.

Using Feedback to Check the Meaning of the Message

Predicting how a person will translate a particular message or understanding a person's background is difficult. Many communication misunderstandings can be alleviated by using a technique described earlier: providing feedback to check the meaning of the message. As senders of messages we should ask others to share their interpretation of the message. In the antibiotic example, the pharmacist should have asked the mother in a nonthreatening manner how long she was going to give the medication. We typically do not ask for feedback from patrons to check their perceptions of the meaning of our messages. Verifying the fact that the receiver interpreted the intended meaning of our verbal and nonverbal messages takes additional time and is sometimes awkward. In addition, most people rely on their own intuition as to whether their intended message was received correctly.

In the potassium example, the pharmacist who dispensed the original medication should have asked the patient to repeat how she intended to take the medication. Thus, the initial perception could have been corrected, and the problem could have been avoided. Examples of how to ask for feedback include:

"How do you intend to take the medication?"

"It is important that I understand that you know how to take this medication. Now when you get home, how are you going to take this medication?"

"Describe in your own words how you are going to take this medication."

The preceding paragraphs describe ways to minimize misunderstanding from the sender's perspective. However, the receiver can also alleviate some misunderstanding by offering feedback to the sender. After receiving the message, the receiver should indicate in some way what she understands the message to be. In later chapters, specific skills will be offered as means to improve your ability to give feedback and receive feedback from others.

TOWARD THE IMPROVEMENT OF COMMUNICATION

This chapter has presented elements of interpersonal communication and has outlined some strategies to improve communication skills. The discussion of improvement implies that behaviors that inhibit communication must be altered. When attempting to change communication behaviors, it is important to place these potential behavior changes in relation to two other concepts: awareness and attitude. As illustrated by Figure 1-2, a change in behavior is frequently built on appropriate awareness and attitudes that are conducive to potential behavior change.

If you hope to develop new behavior, you must increase awareness of your present behavior and also change your attitude toward interacting with others. Awareness of the communication process centers on two important concepts: self-awareness and process awareness.

Self-awareness is the process of recognizing how you actually communicate with others using both verbal and nonverbal messages. It is the process of analyzing how you are communicating at the actual time of the interaction. Part of this process is asking questions such as "What type of nonverbal messages am I sending?" and "Am I using the correct terminology for this patient?" To enhance their own self-awareness, some pharmacists have videotaped themselves in their actual practice settings. In some situations, pharmacists have also had these tapes critiqued by other people, such as fellow staff, administrators, or communications faculty. This process tends to make people aware of their strengths and weaknesses in this important area.

Process awareness involves analyzing the communication process itself while it is occurring. You have to ask yourself, "Is the conversation going in the direction it should go?" "Am I talking too much?" "Are we getting sidetracked?" If the interaction is not proceeding in the desired direction, then you must tactfully move the interaction towards that direction by using some of the com-

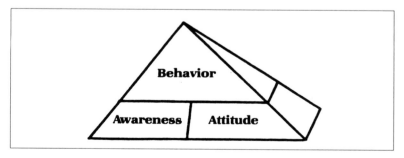

Fig. 1–2. A model for improving communication.

munication skills discussed in this book.

It is well known that those persons who have initiated behavioral changes have taken a good introspective look at their present behavior and have at the same time developed the attitude that good or improved communication is important. When effective communication techniques are achieved, they yield benefits of better patient rapport, more accurate information, optimal patient therapies, greater job satisfaction, and less waste arising from misunderstanding.

SUMMARY

The interpersonal communication model reveals that, as a pharmacist, you need to recognize that interpersonal communication is more than merely speaking, typing a prescription label, or affixing an auxiliary label to a prescription. You need to make sure that the messages you transmit to others are received accurately. There is no guarantee that the meaning of your message will be translated as intended.

In the remaining chapters, we have provided practical skills necessary for you to improve your communication. Each chapter builds on the one preceding it, and the sequencing is deliberate. We trust we can demonstrate that communication is a complex process that may be difficult for some. However, it is a process that can be easily managed and controlled like any other learned skill. By emphasizing practical applications we hope to lower any barriers the reader may have to improvement of a valuable skill.

RECOMMENDED READINGS

Adelman DN: Techniques to improve patient communication problems. NYSJ Pharm., *1*:15, 1981.

Adler AR: *Communicating at Work.* New York: Random House, 1986.

Beardsley RS: How to establish better communication links. US Pharm., *11*:1, 1986.

Berko RM, Wolvin AD, and Wolvin DR: *Communicating: A Social and Career Focus.* Boston: Houghton Mifflin, 1989.

Borman EG, and Borman NC: *Effective Small Group Communication.* Minneapolis: Gordon Press, 1986.

DeVito JA: *The Interpersonal Communication Book.* New York: Harper & Row, 1980.

Dickenson JG: How pharmacists relate to other health professionals. Drug Topics, *125*:28, 1981.

Dunn E: The patient is talking: is the pharmacist listening? Pharmacy Times, *54*:11, 1988.

Eriksen K: *Communication Skills for the Human Services.* Reston, VA: Reston Publishing Co., 1979.

Meadows RJ: Communicating new drug information. Drug Inf. J., *15*:11, 1981.

Pillow WF, and Schlegel JF: Training future communicators. Am. Pharm., *NS21*:43, 1981.

Robinson AJ, and Pillow WF: Communication skills for your pharmacy and community. N.A.R.D.J., *103*:47, 1981.

Russell CG, Wilcox EM, and Hicks CI: *Interpersonal Communication in Pharmacy: An Interactionalist Approach.* New York: Appleton-Century-Croft, 1982.

Srnka QM: Community pharmacy: advisor consultant. Tenn. Pharm., *16*:6, 1980.

Taubman AH, and Matlea EJ: Patient medication intervention program. Am. J. Pharm. Educ., *49*:1, 1985.

Taylor A, Rose Grant T, Mayer A, and Samples BT: *Communications.* 4th ed. Englewood Cliffs, NJ: Prentice-Hall, 1986.

Ver Derber RS, and Ver Derber KS: *Interact: Using Interpersonal Communication Skills.* Belmont, CA: Wadsworth, 1989.

Williams P: *The Vital Network.* Westport, CT: Greenwood Press, 1978.

CHAPTER *2*

Perception and Communication

The Importance of Perception

Sharing the Same Perceptions

Using Feedback to Check Perceptions

Perception, Credibility, and Persuasion

OVERVIEW

This chapter discusses the importance of perception in the interpersonal communication process. People interpret messages based on their perception of the message and of the individual sending the message. Perceptual barriers exist which need to be minimized. Recognizing these barriers and using feedback are skills that are presented in this chapter to enhance your ability to grasp the true meaning of messages.

THE IMPORTANCE OF PERCEPTION

Perception is one of the most important elements in the communication process. As described in the first chapter, interpersonal communication involves the transmission of a message from the sender to the receiver. A critical component of this process is how these messages are interpreted by the receiver. The sender delivers the message, but the receiver may or may not interpret its meaning in the same way the sender intended. The receiver determines the meaning based on his perception of the message and of the individual sending the message.

Perception of Meaning of Message

People assign meaning to verbal and nonverbal messages based on their perception of the intended meaning (Fabun, 1986). In other words, the receiver's perception of the words, symbols, and nonverbal elements used by the sender influences how the receiver interprets the meaning. It is not what is said, but what the receiver perceives to have been said. The following actual situation illustrates this point:

A patient returned to the pharmacy complaining of side effects apparently caused by his medication. The patient's records indicated he had been dispensed 30 nitroglycerin patches. Both the pharmacist and physician told him to "apply one daily." The patient opened his shirt to reveal 27 nitro patches. He perceived the phrase "apply one daily" as an absolute, with no idea of the reality that an old one should be removed before a new one was applied.

The meaning that he assigned to those words was not the same as that intended by the pharmacist. Situations like this occur frequently in pharmacy practice. Many are relatively harmless, but some can be quite serious.

> A young woman suffering vaginal candidiasis was given the usual 15 nystatin vaginal tablets and was told by the pharmacist to "use one daily for two weeks.." She returned to her physician after two weeks in severe discomfort and a complaint that "those tablets taste terrible!" In this example the patient perceived the tablets as being nothing more than regular oral antibiotics and assigned a wrong meaning to the word "use."

Preventing incorrect perceptions like those given above is often difficult because people with whom you interact may have different perceptions about the messages you transmit. Unfortunately, these differences may influence how they interpret messages. In general, people develop their perceptions based on their background, values, and experiences. If we have different backgrounds, values, and experiences, we may assign meanings to messages that are different than those intended by the sender. We are generally unaware of this process, and it takes skill to realize when we have different perceptions from those with whom we are trying to communicate.

Perception of Individuals

Our perception of the message is also influenced by our perception of the individual sending the message (Keltner, 1970). How we perceive the sender affects the interpretation of the message. We respond using our perception of that individual as our reference point. The following story, which has become known as the "Dr. Fox Lecture," illustrates this point.

> Two groups of practitioners were asked to rate the quality of a lecture given on a particular clinical issue. One group of practitioners received a lecture attributed to an officer of impeccable credentials from one of the best-ranked national associations. Another group was given the same lecture but was told that it

was the work of a peer. Practitioners in the first group were apparently mesmerized, although the lecture was delivered identically by the same person. Here one's perception of the message was directly related to one's image of the person sending the message.

We are often influenced by our perception of a person's cultural background, socioeconomic status, gender, or age. These perceptions are influenced by our stereotypes of certain groups of individuals. The following statements illustrate this point.

"Nurses always complain about pharmacists."

"Elderly people can't hear well and always talk too much."

"People who talk slow are ignorant."

We do not see the person as a unique individual but as a representative of a particular group (e.g., elderly, poor, or mentally ill). We erect "perceptual barriers" to the communication process not based on fact but on our inferences. These barriers inhibit true communication between individuals.

It is important to realize that in our normal interactions with others we create perceptions of individuals and make various assumptions. For example, we tend to believe that our patients can speak English unless they tell us otherwise. Unfortunately, this is not always the case because many patients to avoid embarrassment will not indicate that they do not understand. We need to evaluate when our perception of the sender is incorrect, or when our assumptions might be interfering with our ability to communicate with others. Many times we need to "check" our assumption before proceeding further. Does the elderly person really have a hearing deficiency? Does the person who talks slowly have a learning disability? Increased awareness of stereotyping and additional effort in checking our assumptions can enhance our interpersonal communication.

Unfortunately, people we deal with on a daily basis may have perceptions of pharmacists that interfere with our ability to communicate with them. Their perceptions may not be based on reality but on their stereotypes of pharmacists. For example, patient perceptions are influenced by their past experiences with pharmacists, by what others have said about pharmacists, or by what they read in magazines and newspapers. They may perceive us to be uncaring, busy people who are only concerned with filling prescriptions and taking their money. These stereotypes influence what they say to us and how they listen to us. If they perceive us as professionals, they will listen to what we tell them about their medications. By the same token, if nurses, physicians, and other health care providers do not perceive us as professionals, they will not value the information we provide. Part of improving communication with others is to determine what their perceptions of pharmacists are and then try to alter those perceptions if they are unfounded.

SHARING THE SAME PERCEPTIONS

One key to preventing misunderstanding is to try to understand and share the perceptions of other individuals (Applebaum, et al., 1985). Many times, understanding can be enhanced by using "lay language" that is familiar to patients, rather than using medical terminology that is only familiar to health care professionals. Determining the patient's past experience with drugs in general and the particular drugs prescribed may also be helpful. If patients have had positive experiences previously, then they may be more receptive to learning more about the medication. However, if past experiences have been bad, then they may have negative feelings and may be reluctant to discuss or even take the medication.

Frequently, it is difficult to understand patient backgrounds and to predict perceptions of the messages we provide. Some of the skills discussed in the chapter on empathic listening may be of assistance. In many communication interactions, the more we can know about the other individual and the more they can know about us, the easier it is for us to share the same perception.

USING FEEDBACK TO CHECK PERCEPTIONS

A technique that may alleviate some communication misunderstandings is using feedback to check the perceived meaning of the message. As senders of messages we should ask others to share their interpretations of the message. In the nitroglycerin example, the pharmacist should have asked the patient in a nonthreatening manner how long he was going to use the patches. We typically do not ask for feedback from patrons to check their perceptions of the meaning of directions. Verifying the fact that the receiver interpreted the intended meaning of our verbal and nonverbal messages is often difficult because verification takes time and is sometimes awkward. In addition, most people rely on their own intuition whether their intended message was received correctly.

In the second example, the pharmacist should have asked the patient to repeat how she intended to use the medication. Thus, the initial perception could have been corrected and the problem could have been avoided. Examples of how to ask for feedback are included in Chapter 1 and Chapter 8.

The preceding paragraphs describe ways to minimize misunderstanding from the sender's perspective. However, the receiver can also alleviate some misunderstanding by offering feedback to the sender. After receiving the message, receivers should indicate in some way what they understood the message to be. In later chapters, specific skills will be offered to improve our ability to give feedback and receive feedback from others.

PERCEPTION, CREDIBILITY, AND PERSUASION

In many situations, pharmacists need to influence the decisions of patients, physicians, and others. A pharmacist may need to convince a patient that he must take the full 10-day course of antibiotics, or a Pharmacy & Therapeutics Committee in a hospital to delete a certain drug from the formulary. In the search to find the variable that makes one person more persuasive than another, research points to only one factor — perceived credibility. People are influenced by those they believe credible. In the example mentioned earlier, where the same speech was attributed to either a pharmacy student or to an officer of a national pharmacy organization, public opinion favored the national officer. The speech of the national officer resulted in a greater shift in the attitude of the audience, who believed they were listening to the most credible person available. Therefore, being perceived as credible will enhance our ability to be persuasive more than spending hours polishing an impressive style.

What constitutes the perception of credibility? There is agreement that perceived credibility is the combination of three factors:

1.   A safety or trustworthiness element

2.   An expertness or qualifications element

3.   A personal or dynamism element

The trustworthiness factor is a subjective response to the warmth, friendliness, ethics, sociability, fairness, and other factors that enhance the perception of someone being "safe" to talk to. This element is important when conversation requires little or no expertise. Thus, pharmacists who are trusted may find patients asking advice on non-health matters such as personal finance, relationships, buying a car, choosing a college, or any number of subjects.

The expertness factor involves a perception about the competence or education of a sender. It is a factor independent of the other two. One could be labeled trustworthy and highly personable, but sadly lacking in expertise. Naturally, we wish to be perceived as competent by all those who seek our advice. As the public will subjectively evaluate any and all behavior that relates to competency, it behooves us to engage in activities that promote competence, such as displaying awards, certificates, diplomas, and licenses; giving public service talks when asked; seeking and holding office in professional societies; and taking every opportunity to explain what it is that makes a pharmacist a valued member of society.

The personal dynamism factor relates to overall personal characteristics of the sender as perceived by the receiver. For instance, if a pharmacist who counsels a patient for the first time happens to stutter, is slow to respond, and is quite shy, then his credibility may be ranked low despite his great credentials and high knowledge base. However, as subsequent interviews occur, initial judgments may fade if the pharmacist can demonstrate trustworthiness and expertness once the patient gets to know him.

In reality, our interpersonal credibility results from the perception our clientele has of our trustworthiness, competence, and personal dynamism. Before reading further, pause for a moment and ask yourself the following:

1.   How do I believe my credibility is perceived by my patients?

2.   What can I do if I believe my trustworthiness or competence are rated low?

3.   Do I have any personal traits or habits that keep my patients from getting to perceive the real "me"?

SUMMARY

The meaning of the message is influenced by the receiver's perception of the intended message and of the individual sending the message. The following saying summarizes this dilemma:

> "I know that you believe you understand what you think I said, but I'm not sure you realize what you heard is not what I meant."

Thus, it is important to remember the following points when communicating with others:

1.   Anticipate different perceptions in the communication process.

2.   Try to be aware of your stereotypes that may influence your perception of others and be aware of stereotypes others may have of you.

3.   Ask for feedback from the receiver about your intended message.

4.   Provide feedback to the sender to check your perception of the message and to make sure you understood correctly.

5.   Evaluate your level of trustworthiness, competence, and personal dynamism as perceived by others.

REFERENCES

Applebaum RL, Jenson DO, Caroll R: *Speech Communication*. New York: MacMillan, 1985.

Fabun D: *Communications: The Transfer of Meaning*. Toronto: Glencoe Press, 1986.

Keltner SW: *Interpersonal Speech Communication: Elements and Structures*. Belmont, CA: Wadsworth Publishing Co., 1970.

CHAPTER *3*

Nonverbal Communication in Pharmacy

Nonverbal vs. Verbal Communication

Elements of Nonverbal Communication

Detecting Nonverbal Cues in Others

Overcoming Distracting Nonverbal Factors

OVERVIEW

The process of interpersonal communication involves both verbal and nonverbal expression, which includes kinesics, proxemics, and the physical environment in which it takes place. This chapter introduces the components of nonverbal communication and discusses how each plays a part in patient-centered communication.

A large measure of how we relate to others and how they relate to us is not based on what is said, but on what is not said. We need not speak or even have the desire to communicate to be engaged in a communication process. We are constantly providing "messages" to those around us by our dress, facial expression, body movements, and other aspects of our appearance and behavior.

NONVERBAL VS. VERBAL COMMUNICATION

Nonverbal communication involves a complete mix of behaviors, psychological responses, and environmental interactions through which we consciously and unconsciously relate to another person. It differs from verbal communication in that the medium of exchange is not necessarily vocalized language or the written word. The importance of nonverbal communication is underlined by the findings of behavioral scientists, who have reported that 55-95% of all that we communicate can be attributed to nonverbal sources (Mehrabian, 1971; Poytos, 1983). Awareness and skilled use of our nonverbal abilities can make the difference between fulfilling, successful interpersonal relations and frustrated, nonproductive interactions.

Nonverbal communications are unique for two reasons. First, they mirror innermost thoughts and feelings. This mirror effect is constantly at work, whether or not we are conscious of its occurrence. Second, nonverbal communication is difficult, if not impossible, to "fake" in order to have it fit a verbal communication in which we may be involved. Lack of congruence between our verbal and nonverbal messages often results in less than successful interpersonal communication (Borman, et al., 1969).

Nonverbal communication is similar to verbal communication in that each person perceives and interprets a given nonverbal message or "cue" in a totally personal manner. While certain non-verbal "cues," such as a smile, would generally be interpreted to mean happiness by most persons, other nonverbal cues lend themselves to numerous interpretations. This divergence of interpretation stems from the variety of social, psychological, economic, cultural, and other background variables found throughout the human race. Therefore, nonverbal "cues" can and often will have multiple interpretations. However, within a given society, groups of nonverbal cues, "cue clusters," generally provide an interpretation that is universally agreed on. Cue clusters are combinations of nonverbal acts that when taken as a group signify a certain meaning or communicate a certain message. For example, a patient who gives you a friendly handshake, a pleasant-sounding "thank you," and a warm smile at the end of your interaction is probably more pleased with the interaction than a patient who abruptly turns around and quickly walks away mumbling something under her breath. These cue clusters contribute significantly to what is being communicated nonverbally.

ELEMENTS OF NONVERBAL COMMUNICATION

Important nonverbal elements to be discussed in this chapter include kinesics, or body movement; proxemics, or the distance between persons when they communicate; the physical environment; and potential distracting nonverbal elements.

Kinesics

The manner in which you use your arms, legs, hands, head, face, and torso may have a dramatic impact on the message you send. The phrase "turning your back on someone" illustrates this concept well. Down through the ages, societies have developed and refined numerous body movements to communicate certain messages. In this country, for example, it is common for two men who meet to shake hands, and although we are now seeing numerous variations on this basic act, a handshake is a way by which we nonverbally indicate friendship or at least tolerance of another person. The handshake stems from much earlier times, when a man who extended his hand to another was communicating the fact that he held no weapon to do harm to the other. Many of our common nonverbal acts stem from earlier times. The current meaning of these acts may, in fact, bear little resemblance to their initial meanings.

What is common among health professionals is their purpose of serving others. This role dictates that the health professional try to generate a feeling of empathy and commitment to the helping of others. It is apparent, therefore, that your body movement or kinesics should complement this role. Sincerity, respect, and empathy for another person can be nonverbally communicated by an "open" cue cluster. The classic example of an open posture is standing (or sitting) with a full frontal appearance to the person with whom you are interacting. As an open communicator, you should also have your legs comfortably apart, not crossed, arms at the side with the palms of the hands facing front, and a facial expression that expresses interest and a desire to listen as well as speak.

A closed posture, one that would not lend itself to continued communication, occurs when you have your arms folded in front of your chest, legs crossed at the knees, head facing downward, and eyes looking at the floor. If this posture is retained throughout the interaction, or if it suddenly appears during a conversation, the second party may either respond in a similar manner or break off the interaction. Communication from a closed posture may shorten or halt further productive interaction between parties.

You should be aware of your own tendency to close off communication through nonverbal communication. While the closed posture should not be taken as a totally negative act, always to be avoided, it does have the power to halt interactions and should be used appropriately. For example, if during a consultation with sincere intent you suddenly have the impression that the patient is no longer listening or has retreated from the interaction, you should examine your nonverbal communication to see if it is in fact the cause of the disruption.

A list of ways to communicate from an open posture includes the following.

1.   Varied eye contact (consistent, but not a stare)

2.   Relaxed posture

3.   Appropriate, comfortable gestures

4.   Frontal appearance (shoulders square to other person)

5.   Slight lean toward the other person

6.   Erect body position (head up, shoulders back)

Proxemics

The distance between two interacting persons plays an important role in the content of what is communicated. Proxemics, the structure and use of space, is a powerful nonverbal communication tool. Behavioral scientists have found that at different distances between communicators different communications normally transpire (Keltner, 1970). The most protected space is that from full contact to approximately 18 inches from our bodies. We reserve this space for others with whom we have close, intimate relationships. When a stranger, or even a non-intimate associate, ventures into this space during a conversation we experience anxiety and perhaps anger at the trespass of our intimate zone.

A crowded elevator is the best illustration of our need to maintain our intimate space free of strangers. People in a crowded elevator will do almost anything (to the point of standing like statues) to avoid touching one another. If by chance two people in this situation do have bodily contact, they usually make profuse apologies, even though neither person may have had an opportunity to avoid the trespass of space.

We are much more comfortable in our daily interactions when we maintain a distance of 18 inches to 48 inches between ourselves and others. At this distance, casual personal conversations normally take place in our society. Normally the distance maintained between two people engaged in a social or consultative interaction is between 4 feet and 12 feet. In our society, this is the range of distance in which the bulk of our interactions exist. Interpersonal distances greater than 12 feet are generally reserved for those occasions when one person is speaking and others are the audience. This distance allows the speaker to use her voice's maximum capability and implies that little or no interruption from the audience will occur.

You may want to consider the factor of distance whenever you consult with patients. A pharmacist who persists in trespassing into a patient's intimate zone risks appearing bullish and inconsiderate. Therefore, when counseling a patient it is important to stand close enough to ensure privacy, yet at the same time to provide enough room for each person to feel comfortable. Most of the time people do indicate nonverbally whether they feel comfortable with the speaking distance by stepping back or leaning forward.

You should also be aware of interacting at distances that are inappropriate for the nature of the conversation. If you attempt to explain the usage of a rectal or vaginal medication at a public distance you risk embarrassing the patient and may lose the patient's further patronage. Ideally, the pharmacy should have an area set aside for the purpose of consultation. Privacy can thereby be maintained, and you can be assured that the proxemic factor is accounted for in the best possible manner.

Environmental Nonverbal Factors

A private consulting area is an aid in controlling the distance between you and your patients. A number of environmental factors play an important role in the total nonverbal message sent to patients. The colors used in the pharmacy's decor, the lighting, and the use of space in the pharmacy have all been well documented as important nonverbal communication channels (Beardsley, et al., 1977). Perhaps the most discussed environmental factor of the typical pharmacy's design is its prescription counter. It has been described as a barrier to be overcome in your efforts to communicate with your patients. It has afforded those pharmacists who fear interpersonal communications a protective device whereby pharmacist-patient interactions are limited and placed under the full control of the pharmacist. Assuming that we all have a degree of communication apprehension, but we also possess an equal desire to serve to the best of our ability, it is important to recognize that, although the prescription counter serves a utilitarian purpose, it is not the Great Wall of China. When you step from behind the counter, you take a giant step towards communicating interest, respect, and the desire to truly serve the patient.

The general appearance of the pharmacy also plays an important role in conveying nonverbally that you are a professional, skilled at what you do, and sincerely interested in serving your patrons. Dirt, clutter, and a general untidiness in any business carry a negative nonverbal message.

Just as a sloppy, unkempt pharmacy projects a negative nonverbal message, so too does a sloppy, unkempt appearance of the pharmacy's employees. Physical characteristics differ. Most of them are obtained at birth and change little except for the process of maturation and aging; thus you more or less must remain content with them. This fact, however, should not stop you from using clothing and personal appearance to the best nonverbal communication advantage. A professional should dress appropriately. While you want to convey a friendly appearance, you also want to convey assertiveness and professional competence. Your dress has a great impact on how well you accomplish these goals.

Most pharmacists would be dismayed to learn that after a long, skillfully presented patient consultation, the patient left with little knowledge about her drug therapy, but with a distinct remembrance of the pharmacist's dirty jacket or unruly hair. Your appearance and your fellow employees' appearance can complement or destroy all other nonverbal efforts to communicate professionalism, competence, and assertiveness.

Distracting Nonverbal Communication

As discussed in Chapter 1, communication consists of the transmission of both nonverbal and verbal messages in an environment plagued with barriers. An initial step in improving the communication process is to become aware of those barriers. Some of the more common nonverbal barriers are discussed below.

One of the most obvious barriers in nonverbal communication is lack of eye contact with the patient. It is frustrating to talk to somebody who is not looking at you. Unfortunately, many pharmacists unconsciously do not look at patients when talking to them. Their tendency is to look at the prescription, the prescription container, or other objects while talking. This behavior could indicate to the patient that you are not really confident about what you are saying or that you do not really care about the situation. Not looking at the patient also limits your ability to assess how the information is affecting that person, or, in other words, limits you ability to receive feedback from the patient. For instance, does the patient have a questioning look? an expression of surprise? an expression of contentment? As will be discussed in Chapter 5, good eye contact is essential in effective listening. If you do not look the person in the eye, she might get the impression that you are not interested in what she is saying, and thus might not feel comfortable communicating with you. Using good eye contact does not actually mean that you continually stare at the person, but that you spend most of the time looking directly at her.

Another potential distracting nonverbal element is facial expression. You may be sending a message that you may not intend to transmit. For example, you may be communicating a feeling of lack of interest or concern if your eyes continue to move around while talking or listening to another person. This is especially damaging when your facial expressions are not consistent with your verbal expressions. For example, if you say to someone, "Go ahead, I am listening, tell me about it." and then appear to be distracted by something else around you, the person may hear that you are interested but perceive that you are not. People will tend to believe your facial message more than your words.

In addition to facial expression, your body position can show a lack of concern or interest. The body position includes your stance in relation to the other person. That is, are you positioned in an open or closed stance? Your body position is also determined by whether you fold your arms, slouch forward, or tilt to one side. Patients read or sense your willingness to talk to them based on their perception of your body position, which can communicate whether you are really prepared to talk with them or you have more important things to do.

Another potential distraction to communication is your tone of voice. People interpret the message not only by what words you use, but also by the kind of voice you use. For example, a comment in a sarcastic or threatening tone of voice will produce a different effect than the same phrase spoken with an empathic tone. An inappropriate tone of voice can upset people and may create an entirely different meaning from the one intended. In an attempt to remove this potential barrier, many pharmacists have recorded their voices to monitor inflection and its effect on communication. Many have found that they sound far different than expected.

DETECTING NONVERBAL CUES IN OTHERS

Up to this point our attention has been focused on you, the pharmacist. Skilled use of nonverbal communication also involves the detection of those nonverbal cues that are provided by others. It would be impossible to list all the potential nonverbal cues that you could observe from the patients you serve. However, a few of the most common cues will be presented in an effort to increase your awareness of the patient's potential for providing important nonverbal messages.

Earlier, it was indicated that even though we may exhibit similar nonverbal behavior, each one of us interprets nonverbal cues in a highly individualistic manner. A part of how we interpret these messages is based on our personal backgrounds. Just as important in our understanding of our interpretive process is our sensory capacity to gather stimuli to be interpreted. A color-blind person would obviously not have the same interpretation of a visual nonverbal cue as would a person with full visual capabilities.

Some elderly and physically ill persons may have limited or impaired sensual capabilities that will influence not only how they perceive your nonverbal and verbal communications, but how they in turn nonverbally communicate. An elderly person who moves closer or puts a hand to her ear when you speak may be nonverbally indicating that she is having difficulty hearing. Hearing aids, glasses, and other similar devices should be considered important nonverbal cues. You should adjust your communication in accord with the messages these nonverbal cues are sending you.

Patients who appear rushed or nervous should be given consideration when you attempt to consult them about their drug therapy. You may have to take steps to put the patient at ease before attempting to consult with her. The patient's nervous state may be a detrimental factor when you consider how much the patient will actually gain from an extended consultation.

As part of the detection process, you need to check your perception of the nonverbal message, because the message that you receive may not have been the message intended by the sender. The following example illustrates this point:

> During his first externship experience in a community pharmacy, a pharmacy student (Jane, let's say) was assigned the task of receiving new prescriptions from patients. Jane wanted to help the patients and was looking forward to the opportunity of talking with them about their problems. One day Mr. Stevens approached the prescription counter to have his prescription for levodopa refilled. Jane, who did not realize that Mr. Stevens had Parkinson's disease, noticed that his hands were shaking a lot and commented, "Oh, I see you are a bit nervous today, Mr. Stevens. What's the matter?" Jane observed a nonverbal message (rapid hand movement) from Mr. Stevens and assigned a wrong (and embarrassing) meaning to it.

Jane should not have jumped to the conclusion based on one nonverbal cue, but should have noticed that Mr. Stevens' head was also moving and that he walked with a shuffled gait characteristic of Parkinson's disease.

OVERCOMING DISTRACTING NONVERBAL FACTORS

As has been mentioned earlier, the first step in improving interpersonal communication is recognizing how you communicate with others. In the nonverbal area, this self-awareness involves constantly being aware of the nonverbal elements that you use. In this area, videotaping yourself is particularly helpful, because it will reveal the positive and negative aspects of your nonverbal communication.

Once you have discovered what aspects you need to change to become more effective, the next step is a difficult one: finding strategies to overcome these distracting elements. Several suggestions have been made earlier on how specific nonverbal elements can be improved. One thing that should be mentioned is that potentially distracting behaviors can be overcome by using different nonverbal elements. For example, if you find that you naturally cross your arms while talking to others, you can overcome the patient's possible perception that you are acting defensively by using other nonverbal elements, such as smiling, a friendly tone of voice, or moving closer to the patient. The total message received by the patient is a combination of all verbal and nonverbal aspects, not just one isolated component. Another example is that if you have a soft voice and you sense that the patient cannot hear you, then you can lean toward the patient, raise your voice, or move the patient into a quieter section of the pharmacy. The key to this process is to recognize first the distracting nonverbal elements and then try to overcome them in some way.

SUMMARY

Nonverbal communication involves the largest part of all that we communicate. It behooves you to concentrate on your own nonverbal communications, as well as the various nonverbal cues provided by others. In this way, you can become a more effective, skilled communicator. Developing an awareness of your own nonverbal messages and detection of nonverbal messages in others is the first step in developing skilled nonverbal communication.

REFERENCES

Beardsley RS, Johnson CA, Wise G: Privacy as a Factor in Patient Counseling. J Am Pharm Assoc, *NS17*:366-368, (June) 1977.

Borman EG, Nichols RG, Howell WS, and Shapiro GL: *Interpersonal Communication in the Modern Organization.* Englewood Cliffs, NJ: Prentice-Hall, 1969.

Keltner JW: *Interpersonal Communication.* Belmont, CA: Wadsworth Publishing Co., 1970.

Mehrabian A: *Silent Messages.* Belmont, CA: Wadsworth Publishing Co., 1971.

Poytos F: *New Perspectives in Nonverbal Communication.* New York: Pergamon Press, 1983.

CHAPTER 4

Barriers in Communication

Environmental Barriers

Personal Barriers

Patient Barriers

Administrative and Financial Barriers

Time Barriers

OVERVIEW

Within the communication process, numerous barriers exist that could potentially disrupt or even eliminate personal interaction. The potential number of barriers in any pharmacy practice setting is so large that it is a wonder that any communication takes place. Communication is hindered by environmental barriers, such as crowded, noisy prescription areas; the personal fears and anxieties of both pharmacists and patients; administrative decisions; and lack of adequate time. Removal of these barriers involves a two-step process: recognizing that the barriers exist and taking appropriate action to overcome them.

Nothing could be more frustrating than to realize that you are not communicating effectively with someone. For example, you want to complain to your car mechanic that your car still does not run right. While you are telling him about your problem, he continues to look at a pile of papers on the counter and to mutter an occasional "uh-huh." You continue to relate in the best way you can the nature and urgency of your problem. However, he rushes over to the phone, papers in hand, and starts talking into the receiver without even looking up. How do you feel? Frustrated? Angry? Confused? Why? Probably because you feel you can't communicate with this person. He is not listening to you.

Although you may not have been in the situation described above, you can probably understand the frustration, anger, and confusion resulting from this lack of communication. Unfortunately, situations in which communication is less than optimal occur frequently. This chapter will focus on communication problems and will deal with potential barriers to the communication process. Removal of these barriers requires a two-stage process: first, being aware that barriers exist; and second, taking the appropriate action to overcome them. To become a more effective communicator it is essential that you realize when you are not communicating with another person and then try to analyze why the communication is not taking place. One or more barriers may be interfering with your communication. As discussed later, the strategy needed to improve the situation might be somewhat complex.

ENVIRONMENTAL BARRIERS

As Chapter 1 has indicated, the communication process involves five essential elements: the sender, the message, barriers, the receiver, and feedback. Interference with any of these essential elements may cause a breakdown in communication. The message must be clearly received and the feedback related in a manner the other person can understand. Distractions related to the environment often interfere with this process; therefore, the environment in which communication takes place is critical. Some environmental barriers are rather obvious; others are more subtle. One of the most obvious barriers is the height of the prescription counter separating the patient from the pharmacist. These prescription counters exist for three primary reasons: 1) they provide an opportunity for patients to identify where the pharmacist is located, 2) they provide the pharmacist the opportunity to look over the store area periodically, and 3) they provide a private area for the pharmacist to work. Unfortunately, in some situations patients cannot see the pharmacist behind these strategically placed partitions or counters. It is difficult for patients to talk with pharmacists they cannot even see. This type of environment may give patients the impression that the pharmacist does not want to talk to them. These counters can also intimidate some patients and inhibit communication because the pharmacist is standing over them. Ideally, you and the patient should both be at eye level, which will remove possible perceptions of superiority.

Crowded, noisy prescription areas also inhibit one-to-one communication (Beardsley, et al., 1977). Many pharmacies tend to have a lot of background noise, such as people talking, cash registers ringing, or music playing. These noises interfere with your ability to communicate with the patient. In addition, other people may be within hearing range of your conversation, which limits the privacy of the interaction. Privacy is especially important when the patient wants to talk about a personal matter. Another subtle barrier is the pharmacist's desire to answer every phone call, which may give the impression that the pharmacist is not willing to talk to the patient.

Privacy does not necessarily mean having a private room, but both the patient and pharmacist must feel that privacy exists. For example, many pharmacists use hanging plants, planters, or dividers to create the feeling that a private conversation area exists away from the regular traffic areas. Efforts to increase privacy are made fairly easily. For example, many pharmacists use body position (turn away from a busy prescription area) to achieve a more private environment. Paying attention to the amount of privacy can do much to create an atmosphere that causes both pharmacist and patient to communicate with ease.

The presence of a clerk or technician who stands between the patient and pharmacist may be another environmental barrier. In many pharmacies, these assistants are needed to receive and hand back prescriptions, operate cash registers, and help with the over-the-counter purchases. Often, if patients need to talk with the pharmacist, they must first mention it to the clerk, who then relays the message to the pharmacist. In some situations, the pharmacist responds to the assistant (rather than to the patient), who

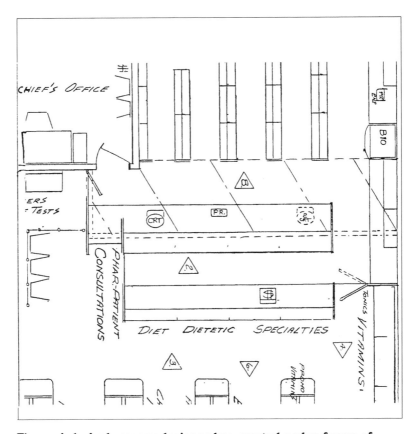

Figure 4–1. A pharmacy designer has created a plan for an effective patient counseling area. (Drawing courtesy of Landon Lovelace Associates, Roanoke, VA)

then passes the answer on to the patient. Obviously, this is not the best method of communication, because both the question and answer can be misinterpreted by any of the three parties. Mechanisms that allow patients to have ready access to the pharmacist need to exist. The clerk must be aware of situations in which the patient truly needs to talk with the pharmacist and must be willing to step aside to allow them to communicate in private. Therefore, as mentioned earlier, your staff needs training in more effective communication as well.

The first step in removing environmental barriers is to find out which ones exist in your practice setting. The best way to do this is to put yourself in the place of the patient. The next time you enter the pharmacy check for the following (see a more complete checklist in the appendix):

Is the pharmacist visible?

Is it easy to get the pharmacist's attention?

Does it appear that the pharmacist wants to talk to patients?

Is the prescription area conducive to private conversation?

Do you have to speak to the pharmacist through a third party?

Is there a lot of background noise or other distractions?

Prescription departments were originally designed to be areas free of traffic so that pharmacists could concentrate on filling prescriptions. Then they were redesigned so that pharmacists could also watch activity within the pharmacy. Today, demands for meaningful patient-pharmacist dialogue require that the pharmacist be accessible and that an area of privacy be offered. For that to happen certain physical barriers must be removed so that the pharmacist has to take as few steps as possible to engage the patient. To accommodate an area for counseling patients, a pharmacy designer should first be consulted to see if it is possible to make a few simple but effective changes in any traditional prescription area, such as the following.

1.   Make countertops wider to accommodate computers and their printer(s).

2.   Place a computer terminal near the patient counseling area to minimize the pharmacist's steps.

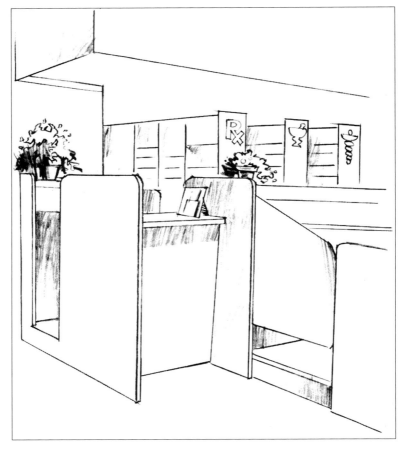

Figure 4-2. By planning ahead for an environment that encourages patients and pharmacists to have face-to-face dialogue, such plans can be translated into a pleasant, efficient and effective pharmacy area.

(Drawing courtesy of Macmillan Healthcare Information)

3. Create a pharmacists-patient interface area that allows easy eye-to-eye contact.

4. Allow a nearby area to be a comfortable waiting area.

PERSONAL BARRIERS

Many personal characteristics can lead to distractions in communication. Lack of confidence in personal communication or low self-esteem may influence how people communicate. People who do not believe that they have the ability to communicate or who are rather shy may avoid talking with others. Many people feel that communication is something you are born with and may use shyness as an excuse not to interact with others. Unfortunately, people do not realize communication skills can be learned and developed, but, like other skills, require practice and reinforcement. Many times reinforcement is not always positive. A negative experience (for example, when a pharmacist has had a fight with a customer and realizes that he did not handle the situation very well) can be damaging to a person's ego and desire to communicate. As with most situations, future performance is based on past experiences — if you have had good experiences you will be more confident when facing future encounters. You need to realize there are no expert communicators and that no one communicates perfectly 100% of the time. Everyone needs to strive for an improvement in communication skills by constant practice.

Another barrier in this area is the degree of personal shyness. Individuals with high shyness levels tend to avoid interpersonal communication in most situations, including interactions in pharmacy practice settings. These people have a high level of fear or anxiety associated with either real or anticipated barriers to communication with others. Overcoming these barriers is a more complex process than overcoming other types of barriers. It requires more time and effort and, many times, professional assistance. However, some techniques, such as systematic desensitization or cognitive modification, have been successful for some persons (Baldwin, et al., 1982). Since these strategies are far too complex to warrant further discussion in this text, we refer you to the counseling literature that discusses these strategies.

One area that is a personal barrier to communication is the internal conversation you may be having within yourself while talking with others. For example, while you are listening to somebody you may be arguing within yourself about whether you want to deal with this person. This internal conversation or "internal monologue" distracts you from listening effectively to another person as you focus your awareness on your own thoughts and arguments rather than on what the other person is saying. Many times these internal conversations result in your prejudging the person and coming to a hasty conclusion or stereotype. Internal messages are essential, because they allow you to sort things out while you are communicating, but they can and do become distracting if allowed to take precedence. It is difficult to recognize that you are more preoccupied with your own thoughts than with listening to the other person. It is essential to develop an awareness of this habit because it can inhibit your ability to listen and can make you appear rude.

Another personal barrier involves the tendency to transfer problems to another person, in this case, patient to pharmacist. In interpersonal communication, it is important to identify ownership of certain problems and associated feelings. Many times, individuals will want to transfer the problem or the feelings accompanying a problem to someone else. They do not want to take responsibility for a problem or the emotional component of the problem. You should realize that if the sender and not you is directly involved with a problem and you cannot personally resolve it, then the sender owns the problem. By the same token, if the sender is clearly the person who is anxious, troubled, angry, or worried, then the sender owns the emotion, not you. If the sender is in an emotional state, you can facilitate communication by using empathic responding to indicate to the sender that you heard his concern. For example, if the owner of a pharmacy discusses his discomfort about using a computer in the pharmacy, the owner (sender of the message) has a problem, not the employee (the receiver). If the listener also becomes uneasy and reacts emotionally, believing that if the pharmacy owner ever acquired a computer then the employee would be the person to run it, then the listener has transferred ownership of the feeling state (the problem) to himself. It might be best for the employee to face his own anxiety and relate it to the pharmacy owner or dissipate this feeling through a third party fairly quickly, before resentment builds up. Emotional objectivity is important in situations in which many people have many problems. As the health care professional, you must attempt to remain empathic but not get so involved that you carry the emotional burden of those with whom you interact. The transferring of other people's problems to oneself is emotionally draining. It is much like losing the charge on a car battery. Eventually it will get to the point where the engine will not start.

Another personal barrier involves cross-cultural factors, which commonly arise when two people from different cultures interact. For example, in some cultures it is not proper to engage in eye contact during communication. From the perspective of these cultures such behavior would be labeled as disrespectful, while in others it would be very appropriate and almost required. Other cultural factors which may limit communication are: 1) different definitions of illness (some patients may not perceive themselves to be ill), 2) perceptions of what to do when ill (some cultures stress self-reliance rather than seeking help), 3) common health-related habits and customs (eating habits), 4) differences in health-seeking behavior (some cultures rely on folk medicine), and 5) perceptions of health care providers (possible distrust of system and possible negative past experiences). It is important to recognize that these and other cultural barriers may exist in the patients which you serve.

Another personal barrier is the fear of being in a situation that is sensitive or difficult to handle. For example, we may not know exactly what to say when a cancer patient expresses fear of dying. Or we may feel awkward when we have to talk to the boss about a sticky personal problem at work. These personal fears or anxieties put tremendous pressure on us to "say the right thing" and may prevent us from talking with others. Often we blow the situation out of proportion; and once the anxiety is confronted and overcome, the actual situation many times turns out better than expected. We are inhibited by our fear of making a mistake.

Another personal barrier is that many pharmacists believe that talking with patients is not a high-priority activity. Many perceive that patients neither expect to nor want to talk with them. It is important to recognize these personal barriers in order to improve interaction. Unlike environmental barriers, removal of these barriers involves personal introspection and analysis of one's motivation and desire to communicate. Removal of these barriers is influenced by pharmacists' ability to change their perceptions. Successful implementation of counseling mandates, such as the Omnibus Budget Reconciliation Act (OBRA) and state regulations, rely on the perception of pharmacists. If they do not value patient interaction, then they will not be as eager to adopt new practices.

PATIENT BARRIERS

The preceding section discussed communication barriers from the pharmacist's perspective. Several variables relate to patients as well. For example, patient perceptions of pharmacists are critical in establishing good communication rapport. If patients perceive us as not being knowledgeable, then they will tend not to ask questions or listen to the advice being offered. Also, if they perceive that we do not want to talk with them, then they will not approach us. On the other hand, if patients perceive us as being knowledgeable and have had positive experiences in the past talking with pharmacists, then they will tend to seek out information. Therefore, we must alter patient perception by first teaching the patient that we sincerely want to communicate with them and then by actually doing it.

Another patient perception that hinders communication is their belief that the health care system is impersonal. Some patients sense that health care providers are not concerned about them as individuals but rather as cases or disease states. They obviously have not been impressed with the empathy displayed by health care givers. You may be seen as a part of this impersonal system. Thus, the perception of impartiality may make patients less willing to talk with you or other health care professionals.

Patient perceptions of their medical condition may also inhibit communication. They often believe that their condition is a relatively minor one requiring no further discussion with you nor other health care personnel beyond the initial physician visit. In contrast, patients may be anxious about their condition and therefore will not talk about it with anybody. Also, many patients share the perception that if a physician has prescribed a medication there is no need to know anything more than what is stated on the label. You need to convince patients that they need to learn about their medications, and you should try to remove some of the patients' inappropriate perceptions about their condition or medications.

ADMINISTRATIVE AND FINANCIAL BARRIERS

Several factors dealing with the administrative or financial aspects of pharmacy practice serve as barriers to communication. For example, pharmacists are not paid directly for educating or communicating with patients; therefore, many managers perceive the task of talking with patients as an expensive service and not a high priority. However, studies have shown that many consumers are willing to pay for such service (Smith, 1983). In addition, research is currently being conducted to document the costs and benefits of patient counseling in an effort to have pharmacists reimbursed by governmental and third-party insurance companies for this valuable service.

Unfortunately, pharmacies have often made policies that discourage pharmacist-patient interaction. Evidence of these policies is often reflected in how certain pharmacy practice settings are organized. High prescription counters, glass partitions, or even bars separating patients from the pharmacist definitely discourage patient-pharmacist interaction. Many pharmacists have limited the number of staff members who can assist pharmacists with their dispensing responsibilities. Shifting workload would allow pharmacists more time to counsel patients.

The mechanics of dispensing prescriptions may distract from the communication process. It is difficult to type a label, count medications, talk on the phone, and complete other necessary dispensing tasks while trying to communicate with the patient. The removal of administrative barriers depends on the willingness of management and staff to alter procedures so that patient interaction can be emphasized. In addition, management must realize that patients who leave one pharmacy and go somewhere else do so because of dissatisfaction with an employee's attitude or with the pharmacy's communication style.

TIME BARRIERS

Choosing an inappropriate time to talk may lead to communication failure. The timing of the interaction is critical, because neither you nor the patient may be ready to communicate at a given time. For example, a woman may have just come from a physician's office where she has waited for three hours with two sick children. The most important thing on her mind is to go home, get her kids to bed, and then relax. She is probably not in the best frame of mind to sit down and have a meaningful conversation with you about the medication. You may also be harried. If a physician is on the phone or a large number of prescriptions need to be filled in a short time, you may feel that this is not a convenient time to talk to the patient. A solution might be to contact the patient by phone or by some other means at a later time, when both you and the patient have a more relaxed period in which to communicate. Many pharmacists have written information that can reinforce a short message during busy situations. Many pharmacists make efficient use of time by using a variety of strategies, such as "highlighting" a patient information leaflet with a highlight pen to emphasize key points. You also need to assess nonverbal messages for assurances that communication is well timed (is the patient really listening?).

SUMMARY

Interpersonal communication, because of its complexity and human involvement, is a fragile process. Messages become helpful to the patient only when they are accurately received and understood. If messages are distorted or incorrect, then they actually may be harmful to the patient and may prevent an effective and meaningful patient outcome. Barriers, such as the ones discussed above, may lead to this distortion. It is important to first recognize potential barriers and then develop a strategy to minimize or remove them.

REFERENCES

Baldwin HJ, Richmond VP, McCroskey JC, Berger BA: The quiet pharmacist. Am Pharm, *NS22*:536, 1982.
Beardsley RS, Johnson CA, and Wise G: Privacy as a factor in patient compliance. J. Am. Pharm. Assoc., *NS17*:366, 1977.
Smith D: Willingness of consumers to pay for pharmacists' clinical services. Am. Pharm., *NS23*:58-64, June, 1983.

RECOMMENDED READINGS

Anonymous: Overcoming barriers to compliance theory and practice. Pharm. J., *235*, Nov. 1986.
Bevlo DK: *The Process of Communication.* New York: Holt, Rinehart & Winston, 1960.
Borman EG, Howell WS, Nichols RG, and Shapiro GL: *Interpersonal Communication in the Modern Organization.* Englewood Cliffs, NJ: Prentice-Hall, 1969.
Dickson WM, and Rodowskas C: Verbal communication of community pharmacists. Med. Care, *13*:486, 1975.
Knapp ML: *Nonverbal Communication in Human Interaction.* 2nd ed. New York: Holt, Rinehart & Winston, 1978.

PART 2

Practical Skills for Pharmacists

CHAPTER *5*

Listening and Empathic Responding

OVERVIEW

Listening to patients — trying to understand their thoughts and feelings — is crucial to effective communication. However, empathic communication requires more than understanding. The understanding you have must be effectively conveyed back to the patient so that she knows you understand. In addition, you must genuinely care about patients and not be afraid to let your concern be communicated. Finally, patients' feelings must be accepted without judgment as to "right" or "wrong." This chapter will examine some of the skills involved in listening and empathic communication. The attitudes essential to empathic communication and the effects of such communication on the pharmacist-patient relationship will also be explored.

LISTENING WELL

When we think about skills of effective communication, we probably think first of the skills involved in speaking clearly and forcefully; in having an effect on others based on what we say. An equally critical part of the communication process, and perhaps the most difficult to learn, is the ability to be a good listener. You have probably experienced a sense of satisfaction and gratitude when you have felt that another person really listened to what you had to say and, to a large extent, understood your meaning. Your ability as a pharmacist to provide your patients and colleagues with this sense of being understood is a crucial part of your effectiveness in communicating with them.

Chapter 1 described the components to the interpersonal communication model and explained the importance of the feedback loop to effective communication. As the receiver of messages, your ability to listen well will determine the accuracy with which you are able to decode messages congruent with the speaker's (patient's) intended message. In addition, your ability to convey your understanding back to the patient will affect the degree to which she feels understood and cared for. If you have failed to understand the patient, this can be uncovered and clarified in the feedback process. If your attempt to listen and understand is genuine, even "missing the mark" will not be damaging if the overall message being conveyed is one of caring and acceptance.

Some communication habits can interfere with your ability to listen well. Trying to do two things at once makes it evident that the patient does not have your full attention. Planning what you will say next interferes with actively trying to understand the meaning of the patient's communication. Jumping to conclusions before a patient has completed her message can lead to only hearing parts of messages — often pieces that fit into preconceived ideas you have. Focusing only on content, judging the person or the message as it is being conveyed, faking interest, communicating in stereotyped ways — all cause us to miss much of the meaning in messages people send us.

Listening well involves understanding both the content of the information being provided and the feelings being conveyed. Skills that are useful in effective listening and empathic responding include summarizing, paraphrasing, nonverbal attending, and reflection of feeling statements that verbally convey your understanding of the essence of another person's communication.

Summarizing

When a patient is providing information, such as during a medication history interview, it is necessary for you to try to summarize the critical pieces of information. Summarizing allows you to be sure you understood accurately all that the patient conveyed and serves as well to allow the patient to add new information that may have been forgotten. Especially when there are barriers in communication, such as language barriers, frequent summary statements serve to identify misunderstandings that may exist.

Paraphrasing

When using this technique, you attempt to convey back to the patient the essence of what she has just said. Paraphrasing condenses aspects of content as well as some superficial recognition of the patient's attitudes or feelings.

The following are examples of paraphrasing:

Patient #1: I don't know about my doctor. One time I go to him and he's as nice as he can be. The next time he's so rude I swear I won't go back again.

Pharmacist #1: He seems to be very inconsistent.

Patient #2: I'm glad I moved into the retirement village. Every day there is something new to do. There are always lots of things going on — I'm never bored.

Pharmacist #2: So there are a lot of activities to choose from.

EMPATHIC RESPONDING

Empathy Defined

Many of the messages patients send to you involve the way they feel about their illnesses or life situations. If you are able to communicate to patients that you understand these feelings, then caring, trusting relationships are established. Communicating that you understand another person's feelings or point of view is a powerful way of establishing rapport and is a necessary ingredient in any helping relationship.

Theoretical Foundations.

The importance of empathy in helping relationships has been elucidated most eloquently by psychologist Carl Rogers. Rogers developed person-centered psychotherapy, which is itself part of a humanistic tradition in psychology (Rogers, 1951, 1957, 1961). Central is the belief that, if people are able to express themselves honestly in an accepting, caring atmosphere, they will naturally make healthy, self-actualizing decisions for themselves. In such an environment, people are able to reach solutions to their emotional problems that are right for them. Others can be helpful primarily by providing a "listening ear" to help the person clarify her feelings. The ability to listen effectively to the emotional meaning in a patient message is the essence of empathy. Empathy conveys understanding in a caring, accepting, nonjudgmental way. The world is perceived from the patient's point of view. Rogers has noted the lack of empathy in most of our communications: "I suspect that each of us has discovered that this kind of understanding is extremely rare. We neither receive it nor offer it with any great frequency. Instead, we offer another type of understanding which is very different, such as 'I understand what is wrong with you' or 'I understand what makes you act that way.' These are the types of understanding which we usually offer and receive — an evaluative understanding from the outside. But when someone understands how it feels and seems to me, without wanting to analyze me or judge me, then I can blossom and grow in that climate" (Rogers, 1967).

The main difference between an empathic response and a paraphrase is that empathy serves primarily as a reflection of the patient's feelings rather than the content of the communication. The following examples, taken from the section on paraphrasing, should illustrate the difference.

Patient #1: I don't know about my doctor. One time I go to him and he's as nice as he can be. The next time he's so rude I swear I won't go back again.

Pharmacist #1: It must be difficult for you to feel comfortable with him if you never know what kind of mood to expect.

Patient #2: I'm so glad I moved into the retirement village. Every day there is something new to do. There are always lots of things going on — I'm never bored.

Pharmacist #2: You really seem to love living there.

In addition to empathy, two other attitudes or messages must be conveyed to the patient if trust is to be established. First, you must be genuine, or sincere, in the relationship. If the patient perceives you as phony, your "caring" a well-practiced facade, then trust will not be established. Being genuine may mean, at times, setting limits in the relationship. For instance, it may be necessary to tell a patient that you do not have time right now to discuss an issue in detail, but will telephone or set an appointment when not so busy. The fact that you were direct and honest about your limits will probably do less to harm the relationship than if you had said, "I'm listening," while nonverbally conveying hurry or impatience. The incongruence or discrepancy between what we say and how we act sets up barriers that are difficult to overcome.

Another essential condition is respect for and acceptance of the patient as an autonomous, worthwhile person. If the pharmacist feels and conveys an ongoing positive feeling for patients, patients can reveal themselves as they really are without fear that they will be judged. They will more likely feel free, for instance, to tell you that they are having trouble with compliance or do not understand directions if they know that you will not think them stupid or incompetent. One of the biggest blocks to effective communication is our tendency to judge each other. If we think that another will judge us negatively, we feel less willing to reveal ourselves. Acceptance and warmth, if genuine, allow patients to feel free to reveal themselves to you.

Empathy and Effective Communication

The positive effects of empathy are many and varied. Empathy helps patients come to trust you as someone who cares about their welfare. It also helps patients understand their own feelings more clearly. Often our concerns and feelings are only vaguely perceived until we begin to talk about them with someone else. In addition, an empathic response facilitates the person's own problem-solving ability. If we are allowed to express our feelings in a safe atmosphere, we begin to feel more in control of them by understanding them better. We also feel freer to explore possible solutions or different ways of coping with our problems.

Put yourself into the role of a community pharmacist. Mr. Raymond is talking with you about his physician. He says: "I've been to Dr. Johnson several times because I heard she was a good doctor. But she just doesn't seem to care. I have to wait for hours even with an appointment. Then when I do get to see her, she rushes in and out so fast I don't have a chance to talk to her. Oh, she's pleasant enough. I just get the feeling she doesn't have time to talk to me."

Which of the following comes closest to being the type of response you might make to Mr. Raymond?

a. "You have to understand that Dr. Johnson is a very busy woman. She probably doesn't mean to be abrupt."

b. "Dr. Johnson is a very good physician. I'm sure she gives patients the best care possible."

c. "I don't blame you for being upset. You shouldn't have to wait that long when you have an appointment."

d. "Tell her how you feel about the way she treats patients. Otherwise, find a different physician."

e. "I'm sure you just happened to see her when she was having a bad day. I bet if you keep going to her, things will improve."

f. "I know how you feel. I hate to wait in doctor's offices, too."

g. "No one feels that they have enough time to talk with their doctors."

h. "How long do you usually have to wait before you get in to see her?"

i. "Let me talk with you about the new prescription you're getting."

j. "You seem to feel there's something missing in your relationship with Dr. Johnson — that there isn't the caring you would like."

Consider the hidden messages you convey to Mr. Raymond with each of the above types of response.

Judging Response

While conveying understanding seems so obviously a part of good communication, a number of less helpful types of response are frequently used in communication with others. Often, for example, we tend to judge another's feelings. We tell patients in various ways that they "shouldn't" feel discouraged or frustrated, that they "shouldn't" worry, that they "shouldn't" question their treatment by other health professionals. Any message from you that indicates you think patients "wrong" or "bad" or that they "shouldn't" feel the way they do will indicate that it is not safe to confide in you. In the example above, responses (a) and (b) indicated the pharmacist thought that Mr. Raymond was "wrong" or that he misperceived the situation. In either case, the judgment was conveyed that he "shouldn't" feel as he does. Even response (c) judges that Mr. Raymond's feelings are "right" and also implies that it is appropriate for you to judge his feelings as "right" or "wrong."

Advising Response

We also tend to give advice. We get so caught up in our role as "expert" or "professional" that we lose sight of the limits of our expertise. We must, as pharmacists, give patients advice on their medication regimens. That is part of our professional responsibility. However, that role is not appropriate in helping a patient deal with emotional or personal problems. The best source of a problem solution resides within the patient. It is presumptuous of us to feel we can offer a quick "solution" to another's personal concerns. In addition, it conveys to patients that we do not perceive them as competent to arrive at their own decisions. Even when the advice is reasonable, it is not a decision that patients have arrived at themselves. Relying on others for advice may keep patients "dependent," seeing others as the source of problem solving. In the example, the pharmacist's advice in response (d) gives a quick (and rather presumptuous) "solution" to what is a complex problem in the eyes of Mr. Raymond.

There are times when patients do want advice and are looking for help with their problems. Assisting them in identifying sources of help they can call on may, at times, be an appropriate way to help patients. Suggesting alternatives for consideration may also be helpful. In this type of response, you are serving as a sounding board for decisions the patient arrives at herself, rather than providing your own solutions.

There are times, of course, when patients are not capable of coping with their own feelings or problems. A typical example is the patient who is severely depressed. Being able to recognize the cues of depression and suggest sources of help, such as the family physician or a local mental health service, is a professional function you must be prepared to perform. However, most people who are ill have feelings of depression and worry that are a normal reaction to the illness. They need to be provided with concerned, empathic care. This empathic concern should be seen as a crucial component in appropriate, humane patient care by all health professionals.

Reassuring Response

A third mode of response to a patient's feelings is a reassuring response. Telling a patient "Don't worry, I'm sure your surgery will turn out just fine" may seem to be helpful, but is really conveying in a subtle way that the person "shouldn't" feel upset. We often use this kind of response to try to get a person to stop feeling upset or to try to change a person's feelings, rather than accepting the feelings as they exist. This type of response may be used even when the patient is facing a situation of real threat, such as a terminal illness. We may feel helpless in such a situation and use false reassurance to protect ourselves from the emotional involvement of listening and understanding the person's feelings. Response (e) is a reassuring response that predicts a positive outcome the pharmacist has no way of knowing will occur.

Generalizing Response

Another way in which we try to reassure patients is by telling them "I've been through the same thing and I've survived." While it is comforting to know that others have had similar experiences, this response may take the focus away from patients and onto the pharmacist before patients have had a chance to talk over their own immediate concerns. It also can lead you to stop listening because you jump to the conclusion that, because you have had an experience similar to the patient's, the patient is feeling the same way you felt. This may not, of course, be true. Response (f) in Mr. Raymond's case would fit in this category.

Response (g) also indicates that Mr. Raymond's feelings are not unique or special in any way. The "everyone feels that way" response, again, is meant to make Mr. Raymond feel better about his problem but instead makes him feel that you do not consider his concerns as being very unique or important.

Probing Response

Another type of response to feelings is a probing response. We feel comfortable asking patients questions — we have learned how to do this in medication history taking and in consultations with patients on over-the-counter drugs. However, asking questions when the patient has expressed a feeling can take the focus away from the feeling and onto the "content" of the message. It also leads to the expectation that if enough information is gathered, then a solution will be forthcoming. Many human problems or emotional concerns are not so easily "solved." Often patients simply need to be able to express their feelings and know that people understand. Meeting those needs is an important part of the helping process. Asking Mr. Raymond how long he has to wait for an appointment — response (h) — does not convey an understanding of the essence of his concern, which was his perception of a lack of caring from his physician.

Distracting Response

Many times we get out of situations we don't know how to respond to by simply changing the subject. With response (i), Mr. Raymond gets no indication from the pharmacist that his concerns have even been heard, let alone understood.

Understanding Response

Contrast each of the other responses to Mr. Raymond with response (j) ("You seem to feel there's something missing in your relationship with Dr. Johnson — that there isn't the caring you would like.") Only in this response is there any indication that the pharmacist truly understands the basis of Mr. Raymond's concern.

The pharmacist conveys this understanding without judging Mr. Raymond as right or wrong, reasonable or unreasonable.

The above discussion reviewed some different responses people tend to make to feeling statements. The following dialogue is an example of a patient-pharmacist communication that may invite quite different responses from different pharmacists. The situation involves Mrs. Raymond, who has come to get a prescription filled for her husband, George. The patient-pharmacist conversation is in the left column, and an analysis of the conversation is in the right column.

DIALOGUE 1

Patient-Pharmacist Conversation	Analysis
Mrs. Raymond: George has been sick so long, sometimes I wonder if he's ever going to get well. I just don't know if I can keep going much longer.	
Pharmacist: Now, of course he's going to get well and you can keep going. You've been so strong about it.	Reassuring or placating response. Mrs. Raymond's reaction to this might be "How can he be so sure George will get well? And he thinks I've been so strong: He has no idea how terrified I've been most of the time."
Mrs. Raymond: But it's taking so long. It seems that Dr. Johnson should be getting George well pretty soon.	Mrs. Raymond seems to be protesting the pharmacist's glib response that she has nothing to worry about.
Pharmacist: Now, you know Dr. Johnson is a good doctor and you shouldn't be questioning her care of your husband. It's important to trust your physician.	Evaluation response. Mrs. Raymond's response to this might be "Of course, he'd stick up for the physician. And it isn't really that. I'm just frustrated and no one understands that."

Patient-Pharmacist Conversation	Analysis
Mrs. Raymond: Well, she's certainly not getting anywhere with George!	
Pharmacist: How long has it been now that George has been sick?	Probing response. Having this bit of information at this point is probably not as important as focusing on Mrs. Raymond's feelings.
Mrs. Raymond: Thirteen months.	
Pharmacist: Sometimes these things take time. Maybe you just need to get away more. I think it would do you good to have someone come in and stay with George, say one day a week, so you can get out more.	Advising response. While this may be helpful, the fact that the pharmacist offered this as a quick solution may outrage Mrs. Raymond. It's as if he can presume to tell her how to cope with the situation when she *has* been coping with it for thirteen months. If anything, she could probably tell him a thing or two about coping.
Mrs. Raymond: I don't want to get out more. I want George to get well.	
Pharmacist: He will, believe me. He is getting the best care possible.	

Contrast the above exchange with the following between the patient and the pharmacist:

DIALOGUE 2

Patient-Pharmacist Conversation	Analysis
Mrs. Raymond: (deep sigh) George has been sick so long, sometimes I wonder if he's ever going to get well. I just don't know if I can keep going much longer.	
Pharmacist: I know it must be very hard on you to see George so ill.	Understanding response. The pharmacist shows that she recognizes the stress that Mrs. Raymond has been under.
Mrs. Raymond: It really is. I sometimes feel that it's hopeless.	Mrs. Raymond confirms that the pharmacist is accurate in her understanding and goes on to reveal a little more about her feelings.
Pharmacist: You seem pretty discouraged right now.	
Mrs. Raymond: (Head nod and nonverbal struggle to control tears).	Often the response to an accurate understanding will not be that Mrs. Raymond will choose to explore feelings further. The fact that someone has listened and understood may be all she needs at the time. The pharmacist lets her decide how much she wishes to reveal by leaving the door open without forcing disclosure through probing.

Pharmacist: (after long pause) Is there something I can do to help?

Mrs. Raymond: Sometimes it helps just to be able to talk to people. Dr. Johnson always tells me not to worry. How can I help but worry?

Pharmacist: It sounds as if people try to cheer you up instead of understanding how difficult it is for you.

Mrs. Raymond: I don't blame Dr. Johnson. I know he's a good doctor. But I'd like her to realize that sometimes I just get frustrated by how long it's taking.

A patient who feels discouraged or angry often needs simply to know that others understand. Mrs. Raymond is not "blaming" you or the physician but is lashing out because of her own frustrations and feelings of helplessness. You do not need to try to placate or judge her feelings (you shouldn't let yourself get discouraged), but you can be helpful by showing concern and understanding.

We try in various ways to get patients to stop or change their feelings. We ourselves may feel uncomfortable in dealing with expressions of emotion, so, to protect ourselves, we cut off a patient's communication. We may try to distract them by changing the subject; we may try to show them things are not as bad as they seem; we may direct the communication to subjects we feel comfortable with, such as medication regimens. These responses, along with numerous others, tend to convey to patients that we are not listening and, perhaps, that we do not *want* to listen. Yet feeling that someone has listened to us and, to a large extent, understood our feelings is a gratifying experience. For a pharmacist, monitoring how well you are listening to patients is as important as carefully choosing the words you use in educating them about their medications.

ATTITUDES UNDERLYING EMPATHY

Underlying empathic responding is an empathic attitude toward others. This attitude means that you want to listen and try to understand people's feelings and points of view. It means you are able to accept feelings as they exist without trying to change them, stop them, or judge them. You are not yourself afraid of a person's emotions and are able to just *be* with a person and not necessarily *do* anything except listen. The empathic person is able to trust that people can cope with their own feelings and problems. If this attitude is held, pharmacists will not be afraid to allow patients to express their feelings and arrive at their own decisions. The empathic person also believes that listening to someone is helpful in and of itself and often is the only means of help one has to offer. Health professionals feel frustrated if they cannot prescribe a medication and "cure" a patient's problems. Yet the emotional concerns a patient brings to you along with her physical problems cannot be "cured" or "treated" in that way. This does not mean that you have no help to provide; it does mean that you must define "helping" in a new way.

In empathic communication, it is not sufficient to feel that you understand another person — empathy also requires effectively conveying to the person that you do, in fact, understand. How can this be done? A response that is effective in conveying that you are listening is to briefly summarize or capsulize what you understand the person's feelings to be. In the conversation between the second pharmacist and Mrs. Raymond, the pharmacist used such a response when she said, "You seem pretty discouraged right now." Such a statement captured the essence of what Mrs. Raymond had been communicating and served to convey to her that the pharmacist had heard and understood her concerns.

The ability to capsulize the essence of the patient's feelings and convey this understanding back to the patient often involves what is called "reflection of feeling." Reflection of feeling has been defined as the statement, in fresh words, of the essential attitudes and feelings expressed by the patient. Reflection of feeling is not simply a repetition of what the patient has said; instead it conveys your attempt to grasp the meaning of the patient's communication in your own words and implies that you are checking to make sure your understanding is accurate. In this sense, the reflection of feeling is not a declarative statement but is tentative and provisional. For example, Mrs. Raymond describes another problem to Ms. Lang, the pharmacist:

"My daughter seems to get sick an awful lot — headaches or nausea and vomiting. I've had her to the doctor but he says there's nothing wrong. I've noticed that she seems to get sick whenever there's a big exam she's supposed to take or a speech she's supposed to give at school. It isn't that I think she's faking, mind you. She really is sick — vomiting and everything."

If Ms. Lang were to respond, "Your daughter seems to get sick a lot — usually right before a big exam at school," she is simply repeating what Mrs. Raymond has told her. Mrs. Raymond might reasonably respond, "That's what I just told you, isn't it?" However, if Ms. Lang were to go beyond the surface meaning of Mrs. Raymond's statement and try to reflect her concern in fresh words, her response might be something like this: "It sounds like you're afraid your daughter may be reacting to the stress she feels at school by becoming physically ill. Is that what you think is happening?"

This response captured Mrs. Raymond's concern but was put into the pharmacist's own words and so was perceived by Mrs. Raymond as showing understanding. In this response, Ms. Lang did not jump to unreasonable or unsupported conclusions about what the problem was. Her response is a tentative "let's see if I understand" kind of response. In addition, she avoided any threatening labels or interpretations such as "You seem to feel your daughter's illnesses are psychosomatic." Such a word would have been too "clinical" and frightening for Mrs. Raymond and would have hindered the pharmacist's attempt to show understanding.

If Ms. Lang had tried to convey her understanding by saying "I know how you feel" or "I understand your concern," the response would not have been as effective as a reflection of feeling response in conveying empathy. "I understand" is a cliché that can be used as a standard response to any feeling statement and thus is not perceived as a response unique to the person with whom you are talking. Because the response also does nothing to convey what your understanding is, it is much less personal and effective than actually trying to reflect the feelings the patient is expressing.

An empathic response implies neither agreement nor disagreement with the perceptions of the patient. If a patient says to you as manager of a pharmacy, "Your clerk was extremely rude to me. She acts as if she doesn't care about your customers," your first impulse may be to check up on the facts. While this is, of course, important and necessary, it does not convey understanding. Your ability to agree or disagree with the patient's perceptions does not help you convey that you understand what those perceptions are. The patient talking to you does not feel cared for, regardless of what the objective truth about the clerk's behavior happens to be.

NONVERBAL ASPECTS OF LISTENING

In conveying your willingness to listen, your nonverbal behavior is at least as important as what you say. As discussed earlier, you can do a number of things to convey your interest and concern. Establishing eye contact while talking to patients, leaning toward them with no physical barriers between you, and having a relaxed posture all help to put the patient at ease and show your concern. Head nods and encouragements to talk are also part of empathic communication. If your tone of voice conveys that you are trying to understand the person's feelings, it, too, complements the verbal message. Establishing a sense of privacy by coming out from behind the counter and getting away from others who may be waiting helps convey your respect for the patient. Conveying that you have time to listen — that you aren't hurried or distracted — makes your concern seem genuine.

Sensitivity to the nonverbal cues of patients is also a necessary part of effective communication. Asking yourself "How is this person feeling?" during the course of a conversation will lead to the discovery that feelings and attitudes are often conveyed most dramatically (sometimes exclusively) through nonverbal channels. A person's tone of voice, facial expression, and body posture all convey messages about feelings. To be empathic, you must "hear" these messages as well as the words that are used.

PROBLEMS IN ESTABLISHING HELPING RELATIONSHIPS

While there are countless sources of problems in interpersonal communication between pharmacists and patients, pharmacist attitudes and behaviors that are particularly damaging in establishing helping relationships with patients include stereotyping, depersonalizing, and controlling.

Stereotyping

Problems in communication may exist because of negative stereotypes health care practitioners hold that affect the quality of their communication. What image comes to mind when you think of the elderly patient? the welfare patient? the AIDS patient? the noncompliant patient? the illiterate patient? the "hypochondriacal" patient? the dying patient? the "psychiatric" patient? Even the label "patient" may create artificial or false expectations of how any individual might behave. Pharmacists who hold certain stereotypes of patients may fail to listen without judgment. In addition, information that confirms the stereotype is perceived while information that fails to confirm it is *not* perceived.

What does the issue of stereotyping mean for pharmacists? First, before pharmacists can be effective in communicating with patients, they must come to know what stereotypes they hold and how these may affect the care they give patients. Pharmacists must then begin to see their patients as individuals with the vast array of individual differences that exist. Only then can we begin to relate to each patient as a person, unique and distinct from all others.

Depersonalizing

There are a number of ways communication with a patient can become depersonalized. If an elderly person is accompanied by an adult child, for example, we may direct the communication to the child and talk about the patient in her presence. We may focus all communication on "problems" and "cases." Discussing only the diseases or the problems a patient has with managing treatment without recognizing or commenting on the successes in treatment, the strides patients make in coping with infirmities, or even the everyday aspects of a patient's life, makes communication narrow and impersonal. A rigid communication format with the process being more pharmacist monologue than pharmacist-patient dialogue can also make communication seem rote and defeat the underlying purpose of the encounter.

Controlling

Numerous studies have found that an individual's sense of control is related to her health and feelings of well-being (Rodin, 1986; Langer, 1983). The construct of sense of control is particularly relevant in examining patient-practitioner relationships (see Schorr and Rodin, 1982, for a description of the theoretical foundation). Interventions to increase levels of patient participation and control in the provider-patient relationship have yielded positive results which include improving clinical and quality-of-life outcomes (Kaplan, Greenfield, et al., 1989). Yet actual communication between health care providers and patients may decrease rather than enhance the perceived personal control of the patient (Schorr & Rodin, 1982). Illness often results in disturbing feelings of helplessness and dependence on health care providers. Added to this patient vulnerability is the unequal power in relationships between providers and patients and the tendency of providers to, all too often, adopt an "authoritarian" style of communicating. Patients are "told" what they should do and what they should not do — decisions are made, often with very little input from the patient on preferences, desires, or concerns about treatment. Yet in the process of carrying out treatment plans, patients do make decisions about their regimens — decisions of which providers remain unaware. Labeling such a patient decision as "noncompliance" is not helpful. Such labeling misses the point that the goal of treatment is to help patients improve health and well-being; it is *not* to get them to do as they are told. Instead of blaming the patient, providers must appreciate the degree to which treatment decisions are inevitably shared decisions. Providers must ensure that information and feedback are conveyed by both providers and patients in a give-and-take process. Providers must actively encourage patients to ask questions and urge them to discuss problems they perceive with treatment, complaints they have about their therapy, or frustrations they feel with progress. This encouragement requires above all else an empathic acceptance of the patient's feelings and perceptions. Patient input is not seen as peripheral to the provision of health care. Instead, the pharmacist must see the patient as the center of the healing process. Establishing a relationship where patients are active participants in making treatment decisions and in assessing treatment effects is crucial to providing quality care.

SUMMARY

Listening well is not a passive process; it takes involvement and effort. It also takes practice to be able to convey understanding in a way that makes it seem natural rather than mechanical or artificial. However, when a relationship between you and a patient is marked by an empathic understanding, the patient is helped in ways medications cannot touch. Patients then experience you as caring for them as persons rather than merely providing care for their illnesses.

REFERENCES

Kaplan SH, Greenfield S, Ware JE Jr: Assessing the effects of physician-patient interactions on the outcomes of chronic disease. Medical Care, 27:S110-S127, 1989.

Langer EJ: *The Psychology of Control.* Beverly Hills, CA: Sage, 1983.

Rodin J: Aging and health: Effects of the sense of control. Science, 233:1271-1276, 1968.

Rogers CB: *Client-Oriented Therapy.* Boston: Houghton-Mifflin, 1951.

Rogers CB: *On Becoming a Person.* Boston: Houghton-Mifflin, 1961.

Rogers CB: The necessary and sufficient conditions of therapeutic personality change. J. Consulting Psychol., 21:95-103, 1957.

Rogers CB: The therapeutic relationship: recent theory and research. In Patterson CH, ed.: The Counselor in the School. New York: McGraw Hill, 1967.

Schorr D, and Rodin J: The role of perceived control in practitioner-patient relationships. In Wills TA, ed.: *Basic Processes in Helping Relationships.* New York: Academic Press, 1982.

RECOMMENDED READINGS

Barnard D, Barr JT, and Schumacher GE: Empathy. In The American Association of Colleges of Pharmacy — Eli Lilly Pharmacy Communication Skills Project. Bethesda, MD: AACP, 1982.

Bernstein L, and Dana RH: Interviewing and the Health Professions. New York: Appleton-Croft, 1970.

Carkhuff RR: Helping and Human Relations: A Primer for Lay and Professional Helpers. New York: Holt, Rinehart & Winston, 1969.

Johnson DW: Reaching Out: Interpersonal Effectiveness and Self- Actualization. Englewood Cliffs, NJ: Prentice-Hall, 1972.

Lawrence GD: If I were in his shoes, how would I feel? J. Am. Pharm. Assoc., 16:453-454, 1976.

CHAPTER *6*

Assertiveness

OVERVIEW

Assertive pharmacists take an active role in patient care. These pharmacists initiate communication with patients rather than waiting to be asked questions. Assertive pharmacists also convey their views of the role pharmacists should play in patient care to other health professionals. Finally, assertive pharmacists try to resolve conflicts with others in a direct manner but in a way that conveys respect for others.

BEGINNING EXERCISE

Before reading further, stop and ask yourself these questions:

1. If a group in your community asks you to give a speech on medication use, do you cringe in horror at the thought of public speaking, and decline the invitation?

2. When a patient is hostile, do you automatically respond with an angry retort?

3. Do patients and physicians you talk with know you by name?

4. Do you make it a point to talk with patients getting a new prescription to make sure they understand their therapy or do you counsel only if they ask questions?

5. Do you look at profile records and ask patients questions on refill visits to make sure medications are being taken appropriately and that there are no problems with therapy?

The questions posed may seem to deal with diverse, unrelated situations — giving speeches, coping with criticism, and counseling patients. Yet they all involve situations where pharmacists can choose to act assertively or nonassertively.

DEFINING ASSERTIVENESS

What is assertiveness? Assertiveness is perhaps best understood by comparing it with two other response styles: passivity and aggression. These three styles of responding are described below.

Passive Behavior

This response is designed to avoid conflict at all cost. The nonassertive person will not say what he really thinks out of fear that others may not agree. The passive person "hides" from people and waits for others to initiate conversation.

Aggressive Behavior

The aggressive person seeks to "win" in conflict situations by dominating or intimidating others. This person promotes his own interests or points of view but is indifferent or hostile to the feelings, thoughts, or needs of others.

Assertive Behavior

This is the direct expression of ideas, opinions, and desires. The intent of assertive behavior is to communicate in an atmosphere of trust. Conflicts that arise are faced and solutions of mutual accord are sought. The assertive individual initiates communication in a way that conveys concern and respect for others.

The critical factor in being assertive is the ability to act in ways that are consistent with the standards we have for our own behavior. When we tell ourselves that other people "make" us feel or act a certain way, we are not taking responsibility for our own behavior. Instead of changing ourselves, we try (impotently) to get others to change. We believe, as Mark Twain noted, that "nothing so needs reform as other people's bad habits." However, the only power we have to effect change in any relationship is to change our own behavior.

Too often, our goals in communication are defined in terms of what we want others to do rather than what we will do. For example, we might say that we want other people to understand what the role of the pharmacist should be instead of saying we will tell others, as clearly and persistently as we can, what we think the role of the pharmacist should be. In addition we will act in accordance with those standards.

If we tell others and show them by our behavior what we want to achieve, many will understand our point of view and some will agree with it. But if they do not agree, it does not mean we have failed or that they should be severely blamed for not understanding. A critical aspect of assertiveness is our ability to respect the rights of others, even when we do not agree with them.

A number of skills are needed for assertive communication. These include: initiating and maintaining conversations, encouraging assertiveness in others, responding appropriately to criticism, giving negative feedback acceptably, expressing appreciation or pleasure, making requests, setting limits or refusing requests, conveying confidence both verbally and nonverbally, and expressing opinions and feelings appropriately.

THEORETICAL FOUNDATIONS

Assertiveness training and theories about how people learn to respond in passive or aggressive ways grow primarily out of cognitive and behaviorist psychological theories. Behaviorists believe that passive or aggressive responses have been reinforced or rewarded and thus strengthened. Aggressive behavior often works in the short term because others feel intimidated and allow the aggressive person to get what he wants. Passive behavior is reinforced when the individual is able to escape or even avoid conflict in relationships and thus escape the anxiety that surrounds these conflicts.

Cognitive theories hold that people respond passively or aggressively because they hold irrational beliefs that interfere with assertiveness. These beliefs involve:

1. fear of rejection or anger from others and need for approval (everyone should like me and approve of what I do),

2. overconcern for the needs and rights of others (I should always try to help others and be nice to them),

3. belief that problems with assertiveness are due to unalterable personality characteristics and are, therefore, unchangeable (this is just how I am), and

4. negative self-evaluation combined with perfectionistic standards (I must be perfectly competent. If I am not, then I am a failure).

Because these beliefs are excessively perfectionistic, they are considered irrational. In the nonassertive person they create anxiety that leads the individual to try (unsuccessfully) to avoid the inevitable conflicts that arise in relationships. These unrealistic standards are also turned on others, leading to angry, aggressive behavior, with frequent "blaming" of others for normal human failings. Cognitive restructuring teaches people to identify self-defeating thoughts that produce anxiety or inappropriate anger in difficult situations and replace them with more reasonable thoughts. As these new thoughts replace the self-defeating thoughts, they begin to be incorporated into the person's belief system. For example, a pharmacist who feels "used" by the boss who always counts on him and only him for emergency coverage might currently say to himself "I don't want to come in to work on my day off this week, but if I say 'no' the boss will get mad and that would be awful." Because this causes him anxiety at the imagined catastrophic consequences of saying "no," he inhibits this response. A more rational thought process when faced with such a request would be "I don't want to work on my day off this week. It is my right to say no. I am not responsible for solving all the problems my manager has in finding back-up coverage." This thought reduces anxiety and frees the person to practice new, more assertive responses to difficult situations.

How do these assertive problems relate to your ability to function more effectively as a pharmacist?

Let us examine some typical situations in pharmacy practice and determine what might be the most assertive way for you to respond in these relationships with patients, physicians, employees, employers, and colleagues.

ASSERTIVENESS AND PATIENTS

Perhaps the most important assertive skill in relating to patients is your willingness to initiate communication. Coming out from behind the counter, introducing yourself, providing information on medications, and assessing the patient's use of medications and problems with therapy distinguishes the assertive pharmacist from the passive one. The passive pharmacist hides behind the counter, gives prescriptions to clerks to hand to patients, and generally avoids interaction with patients unless asked a question. In this way, passive pharmacists are able to avoid the potential conflicts inherent in dealing with people and are able to hide their own feelings of insecurity and fears about being incompetent. While a passive approach may arise out of (or at least be rationalized by) a feeling of time pressure, the passive pharmacist makes no attempt to find alternative ways of providing better patient care, such as giving out medication leaflets and calling the patient during slower evening hours to discuss key points and assess problems. Instead, the passive pharmacist deals with things as they come and takes the path of least resistance in providing minimal (and subprofessional) levels of pharmacy services.

Encouraging patients to be more assertive with you and other health professionals is also an important skill in improving your communication with patients. Helping patients prepare for visits with health professionals and encouraging their active participation in consultations has been found to improve communication and make patients more assertive in their communication (Roter, 1977; Kaplan, et al., 1989). Pharmacists may do this by suggesting that patients keep a list of questions they want to ask during their next visit. Pharmacists may also have patients fill out a brief, open-ended questionnaire when they arrive for a visit in which they write down questions or concerns they have about their health or treatment, information they would like to have provided, or issues they would like to discuss. This process can help patients organize their thoughts and can counteract the passivity patients may adopt in the presence of a health professional. During the visit, pharmacists can actively solicit questions, concerns, and preferences regarding health care. Even normally assertive patients may experience enough anxiety in communication with providers that they forget to ask questions or bring up concerns they have.

A particularly difficult situation that you will face in pharmacy practice is responding to an angry or critical patient. While no one likes to hear criticism, there are ways of dealing with criticism in a rational, assertive manner. When you hear criticism from patients, it is important to keep in mind that the patient's feelings of hostility may be greatly magnified by the life stresses he is experiencing. Patients are usually ill, sometimes seriously ill, and are feeling helpless and dependent on health professionals. They may feel shuffled about, kept waiting in a physician's office, and finally kept waiting for a prescription by a health professional they do not even see except for fleeting moments while the pharmacist moves about behind the prescription counter. It is important, therefore, to keep in mind that some (do not assume all) patient anger arises from frustrations about being ill, and not from personal grievances against you.

When patients are reacting primarily to the stresses of being ill, it is most helpful for you to try to understand what it is like for them and to respond empathically. An empathic response when patients react with shock and dismay at the cost of their medications will probably be more helpful than an attempt to justify the cost. Saying, "You're right. These medications are expensive. Are you worried about whether you can afford them?" shows that you understand the patient's worry and allows you to assess if the concern about cost is a real problem of inability to afford treatment or a way of expressing diverse feelings of frustration.

Another skill that is useful in responding to patient criticism is to get patients to turn criticism into useful feedback. For example, if a patient tells you that your pharmacy does not seem to care about the customer, it is important to find out specifically what is causing the problem. Asking "What specifically is it that upsets you?" may give you feedback that would be useful in improving your pharmacy operation. You now have the information you need in order to decide if you should make changes to improve patient care. Alternatively, you may decide to continue with current policies, but might see the need to better communicate your reasons for these decisions to patients.

ASSERTIVENESS AND PHYSICIANS

When there is a problem in a patient's medication therapy, a consultation with the physician is often required. Even when the problem is one of noncompliance with regimens and you have attempted to intervene directly with the patient, the physician may still need to be apprised of the problem. If you have determined that a phone call is in order and you wish to speak directly with the physician, you will be most effective if you are persistent with receptionists and nurses in your request to speak directly with the physician. Messages transmitted through third parties may not be the most effective means of communication. Such persistence might sound something like this:

Pharmacist (to physician's nurse): This is John Landers, the pharmacist at Central Pharmacy. I'd like to speak to Dr. Stone please.

Nurse: He's with a patient right now. What is it you wish to speak to him about.

Pharmacist: I am concerned about the prescription for Mrs. Raymond for cimetidine. I will need to speak to Dr. Stone about it. Please have him call me as soon as he comes out from the patient examination.

Nurse: It might be quicker if you tell me what the problem is. I could talk to Dr. Stone and get back to you.

Pharmacist: Thank you, but in this case I would like to talk to Dr. Stone directly.

Nurse: He's very busy today and we're running behind schedule.

Pharmacist: I know he has a busy schedule but I must speak with him as soon as possible. Will you ask him to call?

The pharmacist in this communication was assertive. He showed respect for the nurse and yet was persistent in stating his request. He did not argue about the issue of which method of communication was quicker. He calmly restated his request without anger or apology.

Now, let's say you have managed to get through to the physician.

Compare the following introductory comments by a pharmacist.

a.   Dr. Stone, this is the pharmacist at Main Street Pharmacy. I'm sorry to bother you — I know you're busy — but I think there's a problem with Mrs. Raymond's prescription for cimetidine.

b.   Dr. Stone, this is John Landers, the pharmacist at Main Street Pharmacy. I'm calling about a potential problem with Mrs. Raymond's prescription for cimetidine.

In (a), the pharmacist did not introduce himself, which makes him an anonymous employee of a pharmacy rather than a professional with an individual identity. Also, in (a), he subtly "apologizes" for calling, which makes him seem insecure and unassertive.

Here are several ways the pharmacist could proceed:

a.   Mrs. Raymond is already taking diazepam. I don't want to question your decision, but did you know these two drugs can interact? Do you want to change her prescriptions?

b.   Mrs. Raymond is already taking diazepam, and cimetidine can increase blood levels of diazepam. Oxazepam and alprazolam don't present these problems, so you might want to consider switching to one of these.

Response (b) is better. The pharmacist is not putting the physician on the spot by asking him if he knew there was a drug interaction. Instead, he presented the problem that concerned him and suggested alternative medications that would not present a problem.

When identifying potential problems, you should be prepared to identify alternatives to resolve the problem and to make and support your own recommendations. In order to do this with confidence, you should have done the necessary reference reading before making the phone call. Having information on current research "in reserve" in case you need to cite it to convince the physician will increase your effectiveness in making a recommendation. Once you are sure of your facts, it is easier to be persistent in pushing for a therapeutic change that is required. Be sure that you feel prepared to use the medical terms and speak to the physician as a fellow health professional.

You are faced with many barriers to communicating effectively with physicians. Physicians may not accept recommendations and may, in fact, seem ungrateful, if not hostile, to some of your interventions. Even when you do effect a change in physician behavior, you may not receive feedback that your efforts have been effective. Perhaps the next prescription the physician writes will show a change, even though the feedback to you indicated that a change would not be made.

Unfortunately, you are often not going to get a "pat on the back" for consultations with physicians. It is important to keep in mind, therefore, that consulting with physicians if problems arise or asking questions if something seems to be a problem must be done in spite of what the physician's reaction might be. To fail to consult a physician because of anticipated resistance reduces your professional role to one of subservience — one where you are willing to abdicate your responsibilities as a health professional or fail to act in the patient's best interest because you feel uncomfortable carrying out these patient care functions. The assertive pharmacist is aware at all times that his professional duties are to the patient and is assertive (and persistent) in seeing that the best interests of patients and patient rights to appropriate drug therapy are met.

ASSERTIVENESS AND EMPLOYEES

The manager of a hospital outpatient pharmacy has observed lately that one of the pharmacists has been creating problems. The manager's major concern is that the pharmacist is sometimes rude and abrupt with patients. Today, the manager overheard the pharmacist respond with obvious annoyance to a patient who expressed confusion about how to take her medication. The manager decides to talk privately with the pharmacist about his behavior.

"I overheard your conversation with Mrs. Raymond this afternoon when you became impatient with her for not understanding instructions. I was upset because I didn't think you treated her with respect. I want you to treat patients with more courtesy and not get so impatient and judgmental with them."

"Well, she had been complaining about how slow we were and then wouldn't pay attention when I was explaining the directions. I just got fed up."

"I know that patients can be irritating, but I want you to treat them with respect."

"Well, we were so busy then that I just didn't have time to fool around."

"I know it gets hectic and you were feeling rushed today, but even then I want you to be more courteous."

"Well, it would certainly be easier to take time to be nice if you'd get enough pharmacists in here to cover the workload. And if you'd train the techs better, they could be a lot more help to us."

"Those things may be true, but they're beside the point. I want you to agree to treat patients with respect, regardless of how busy we get. Will you do that?"

"That's easier said than done."

"Will you do it?"

The manager of a pharmacy is responsible not only for how he communicates with patients, but also how other pharmacists and supportive personnel treat patients. He must make clear to all employees what he expects in the way of patient care. In the previous scene, the pharmacy manager used a number of assertive techniques in his conversation with the pharmacist. For one thing, he was specific about how he expected the pharmacist to behave and calmly repeated these expectations (called a "broken-record" response) in spite of the pharmacist's excuses. He would not let himself be dragged off the point. He did not become defensive when the pharmacist attacked his performance as a manager. He might also have said, "I would like to discuss any ideas you might have about improving the training of techs another time, but right now I want to talk about the way you counsel patients." This would have let the pharmacist know that he was willing to listen to specific, constructive suggestions but not before the current problem was resolved.

The pharmacy manager also used appropriate feedback techniques. He told the pharmacist what he had observed about a specific behavior and what he wanted changed without attacking the pharmacist as a person. The manager did not label the pharmacist as being rude or thoughtless. Focusing feedback on what a person does is much less destructive than making personal judgments about him as a person. Such feedback also lets him know exactly what must be changed to improve his performance. The manager discussed the situation privately and soon after the incident occurred. Dealing with such a problem immediately is much more effective than waiting until the annual job performance evaluations or until the problem has become so serious that more drastic action is required.

Many of the same guidelines that are useful in giving negative feedback apply as well to praise. A personal statement, such as telling a clerk, "I really appreciate your willingness to stay late tonight to help out" is more meaningful than a general statement like, "You're a good clerk." In addition, if positive feedback is an ongoing part of the relationship rather than something that only gets written on job performance evaluation forms, it is more effective. Too often, employees feel that the only time they get any feedback from their bosses is when they have done something wrong, which makes it much harder to accept the negative comments. Finally, your willingness to accept even negative feedback from employees (if it is constructive) can create an atmosphere of mutual respect. In the example above, the pharmacy manager conveyed both an assertive and empathic message when he said, "I know it gets hectic and you were feeling rushed today, but even then I want you to be more courteous." He let the pharmacist know that he understood the feelings of frustration and at the same time insisted that certain standards be met in patient care.

ASSERTIVENESS AND EMPLOYERS

It is necessary to be assertive not only with your employees, but with your supervisors as well. We often "do as we are told" rather than identifying our goals in communication with supervisors and being persistent in pursuing those goals. As health professionals, we sometimes work in situations where supervisors share neither our professional identities nor the ethical standards we hold for patient care. It is necessary for us, then, to define what the professional standards for pharmacists are and to be assertive in insisting that we must meet those standards whatever our practice environment.

In addition, we may be faced with a situation where we receive a negative evaluation or criticism of our performance by a supervisor. None of us enjoys hearing that someone is angry or disappointed with us for what we have done. Yet the criticisms we receive (and what we do in response to them) can lead to improved relationships with others, if we can avoid some common pitfalls in our responses to criticism.

For some of us, our first response to criticism is to counterattack. The attitude is, "So what if I did make a mistake — I've seen you blow it a few times yourself." It is as if we can somehow "even the score" by criticizing the accuser. However, such a response means we never have to deal with the possibly valid concerns others have about our behavior — we can always change the subject to their problems. In contrast to these aggressive responses, for more passive people, the initial response to criticism is to apologize excessively, give excuses, and generally act as if it is a catastrophe if someone is upset with us. Neither a passive nor aggressive response fosters problem solving.

When you are criticized, it is important to distinguish between the truths people tell you about your behavior and the judgments (the "wrong" or "bad" indictments) that they attach to your behavior. Often these judgments are arbitrary and are based on values you do not share. Even when you do agree with your criticizer and think you were wrong, you must separate the foolish or careless thing you did from yourself as a person. The following are five responses that are helpful in various types of situations where criticism is levied.

Getting Useful Feedback

If the criticism is vague, it is necessary first to find out exactly what happened to lead to the criticism. Uncovering the problem will provide you with feedback that may be useful to you in improving your performance. Therefore, before reacting to any problem that may be present, first be sure you know the exact nature of the problem.

Agreeing with Criticism

If you consider the criticism you receive to be valid, the most straightforward response is to acknowledge the mistake. If it is possible to counteract any of the damage, then that is done. In any case, avoid "Yes, but ..." responses that try to excuse behavior but lead to increased annoyance on the part of the other person. "Yes, I am late for work a lot, but the traffic is so bad" usually leads to an escalation of the conflict ("You'll just have to leave home earlier!"). If you made a mistake or are wrong, acknowledge that without excuses.

Disagreeing with Criticism

Often criticism is not justified or is not appropriate because it is too broad, it is a personal attack rather than a criticism of specific behavior, or it is based on value judgments that you do not agree with. If you consider criticism unfair or unreasonable, it is important to state your disagreement and tell why. For example, you came in late to work this morning and your boss is fuming. During his attack, he says, "You're always late. Nobody around here cares about the patients waiting to get prescriptions filled."

It is important to say to him: "You're right, I was late this morning, and for that I apologize. But it is not true that I am always late. I am seldom late for work. And it is not true that I do not care about our patients. I think the way I practice shows them my concern."

Not to speak up against something you consider to be a personal injustice or untruth leads to feelings of resentment and a loss of self-esteem for having kept quiet.

Fogging

Fogging involves acknowledging the truth or possible truths in what people tell you about yourself while ignoring completely any judgments they might have implied in what they said. Manuel Smith (1975) outlined this as a basic assertive response to criticism. Let us see how this might apply in a pharmacy situation.

Supervisor: You spent a lot of time talking with that patient about a simple OTC choice.

Pharmacist: You're right. I did.

Supervisor: The other pharmacists let clerks do a lot of that sort of stuff.

Pharmacist: You're probably right. They may not spend as much time as I do on OTC consultations.

Such a response allows you to look at possible truths without accepting implied criticisms. The response makes it clear that your own standards for patient care guide your behavior, rather than external judgments you do not agree with.

Delaying a Response

If the criticism takes you by surprise and you are confused about how to respond, give yourself time to think about the problem before responding. Few conflict situations call for an immediate response. If you are too surprised or upset to think clearly about what you want to say, then delay a response. Tell the person: "I want time to think about what you've told me, and then I'd like to sit down with you and try to clear up this problem. Could we get together this afternoon?"

ASSERTIVENESS AND COLLEAGUES

The techniques for assertiveness with employers can also help you be more assertive with your colleagues. For example, the president of your local pharmacy association calls you and asks you to serve as chairman of a new committee. You are interested in the committee but are not sure you have the time. You respond:

a.   "Well, I'd really like to. I don't know. I guess I could if it doesn't take too much time."

b.   "Why don't you ask Jim? He'd be good. Maybe if you can't find anyone else, I could do it."

c.   "I've given enough time to this organization. Everyone always comes to me. Let someone else do some work for a change."

d.   "I'm interested in the committee, but I'm not sure I have time. Let me think about it tonight and I'll call you in the morning with my decision."

Response (d) seems most honest and assertive. We often feel that we must respond immediately to situations. Often the best response is to delay a response. It gives you time to decide what it is you really want to do. When you are facing a decision or when you are embroiled in a conflict, it is often best to say, "I want time to think. I'll get back to you." It is, of course, essential that you do get back to that person when you say you will and resolve the issue. Response (a) is a wishy-washy "yes." The problem with such a response is that you may say "yes" but never really take responsibility for your decision. The "yes" was given because you found it difficult to say "no." Response (b) suggests that, if no one else will do it, you will feel that you must do it. You feel responsible for solving the president's problem by identifying someone to chair the committee. If he cannot find someone else, you will then feel obligated. The aggressive response, (c) is often the point a person comes to after a history of passive responses to similar requests. It sounds as if this person has said "yes" frequently in the past, felt overcommitted, and began to blame others for "asking" rather than taking personal responsibility for having said "yes." It is perfectly all right for others to make requests of you. However, it is up to you to say "yes" or "no" or to set limits on the extent of your involvement.

Let's now imagine a situation where the president tries to coax or manipulate you into changing a "no" to a "yes" response to his request to chair the committee.

President: You would be perfect for the job. It is extremely important and I must have someone who knows the issues and stays on top of things.

Pharmacist: I appreciate that, but I won't be able to chair the committee this year.

President: I'll help with the workload. It shouldn't take more than an hour or so a week.

Pharmacist: That may be true, but I'm not willing to chair the committee right now.

President: Why not? Perhaps there is something we can do to resolve the problems you seem to think will come up in chairing the committee.

Pharmacist: The decision is really a personal one. I won't be able to chair the committee at this time.

In this instance, the pharmacist again used a "broken record" response. He calmly repeated his "no" response without elaboration and with no rancor at the president's efforts to coax him into changing his mind. If the pharmacist had chosen to do so, he might have given an explanation for his decision, but he is not "obliged" to do so. The danger for passive people in giving an explanation is that they seem to believe that the president must agree that the decision is "justified" before they feel they have the right to say "no."

SUMMARY

Assertiveness is a style of response that focuses on resolving conflicts in relationships in an atmosphere of mutual respect. To be assertive, each person must be able to directly and honestly convey "This is what I think." "This is how I feel about the situation." "This is what I want to have happen." "This is what I am willing to do." This type of communication allows all people to stand up for their own rights or what they believe in without infringing on the rights of others. The focus is on problem solving rather than turning the conflict into a "win/lose" situation that damages the relationship.

You as a pharmacist are faced with numerous changes in your role within the health care system. If you are to lead these changes, to have a hand in shaping your own future, then you must be assertive in presenting your own vision of pharmacy's future.

REFERENCES

Kaplan SH, Greenfield S, Ware JE Jr: Assessing the effects of physician-patient interactions on the outcomes of chronic disease. Medical Care, *27*:5110-5127, 1989.

Roter D: Patient participation in patient-provider interactions: The effects of patient question-asking on the quality of interactions, satisfaction and compliance. Health Education Monographs, *5*:281-315, 1977.

Smith M: *When I Say No, I Feel Guilty.* New York: Dial Press, 1975.

RECOMMENDED READINGS

Alden L, and Safran J: Irrational beliefs and nonassertive behavior. Cognitive Therapy and Research, *2*:257-264, 1978.

Ellis A: *Reason and Emotion in Psychotherapy.* New York: Lyle Stuart, 1962.

Heisler G, and Shipley RH: The ABC model of assertive behavior. Behavior Therapy, *8*:509-512, 1977.

Kimberlin CL, Lemberger MA, and Maple MM: Self-assurance in pharmacy practice. In *Lilly Communication Skills Project.* Bethesda, MD: AACP, 1986.

Lazarus AA: *Behavior Therapy and Beyond.* New York: McGraw-Hill, 1971.

Ludwig LD, and Lazarus AA: A cognitive and behavioral approach to the treatment of social inhibition. Psychotherapy: Theory, Research, and Practice, *9*:220, 1978.

McKenzie LC, Kimberlin CL, et al.: *Pharmacists' Care of Elderly Patients.* Gainesville: University of Florida, 1988.

Schwartz RM, and Gottman JM: A task analysis approach to clinical problems: A study of assertive behavior. J. Consulting Clin. Psychol., *44*:910-920, 1976.

Wolfe J, and Lazarus AA: *Behavior Therapy Techniques.* New York: Pergamon Press, 1966.

Wolfe J: *Psychotherapy by Reciprocal Inhibition.* Stanford, CA: Stanford University Press, 1958.

PART 3

Putting It All Together

CHAPTER 7

Interviewing and Assessment

Introduction

Patient Assessment and Educational Diagnosis

Components of an Effective Interview

Interviewing as a Process

Interviewing Using the Telephone

OVERVIEW

Patient assessment is an important aspect of patient care. Determining what patients understand about their medications, how they are taking their medications, and problems they perceive with the therapy are key elements to ensuring positive health outcomes. Gaining insights into patient understanding and actions assists pharmacists in planning an appropriate strategy for increasing understanding and patient compliance. Interviewing is one of the most common methods used in patient assessment. Although it is a common occurrence in pharmacy practice, the patient interview is an area that receives very little attention by pharmacists. This chapter focuses on ways of improving patient assessment and the interviewing process. It addresses aspects of both informal questioning and the more formal, structured interview. Communication skills discussed include questioning, listening, using silence appropriately, and developing rapport.

INTRODUCTION

Pharmacists often need to obtain certain information from patients as part of the patient assessment process. Inquiries range from rather simple requests, such as asking if a patient is allergic to penicillin, to rather complex problems, such as determining if a patient is taking medication properly. At first glance, this process appears to be rather simple; it is something pharmacists do many times each day. However, research and experience have shown that in most cases interviewing is a complex process in need of more attention, because the quality of the information received is not always the best. The following example illustrates this point.

A pharmacist checking for potential drug-drug interactions asked a patient who was starting to receive Coumadin, "Do you take any drugs?" The patient stated emphatically "NO!" The pharmacist proceeded to dispense the medication which the patient took for five days until he visited an emergency room for a nose bleed that would not stop. It was later discovered that the patient had been taking high doses of aspirin for his arthritis. The patient misunderstood the meaning of the term "drugs" and thought the pharmacist was referring to street drugs. Thus, the wrong information was transmitted from the patient to the pharmacist, resulting in a potentially serious drug interaction.

As seen in this example, the accuracy, depth, and breadth of the information provided are influenced by many factors, such as the patient's perception of the interview and the physical environment in which the interview takes place — factors which have been discussed earlier. However, the accuracy of the patient assessment is also influenced by the interviewing process used and the way questions are asked by pharmacists. If the pharmacist in the above example had paid attention to how her question was phrased, she would have found out additional information which would have influenced her course of action.

PATIENT ASSESSMENT AND EDUCATIONAL DIAGNOSIS

The following "educational diagnosis" sequence is provided as one example of a patient assessment process. It places the collection of information in the context of patient education and counseling. To become an effective educator, pharmacists should use the following sequence:

1. Assess what the patient needs to know.

2. Assess what the patient already knows.

3. Identify information gap (between 1 and 2).

4. Assess the patient's ability to learn.

5. Determine the best way to instruct the patient.

6. Determine the best time to instruct the patient.

7. After instruction, assess whether learning occurred.

One of the first steps in this patient assessment process should be to determine what your patients already know about their medications and their health-related problems. Determining how much patients know is necessary because patient education strategies vary depending on the depth of knowledge. Patients who are very familiar with their medications have different needs than those who know relatively little. You become more efficient if you can identify those individuals who need extra counseling. It is very inefficient to repeat information which patients already understand. Using this technique, you essentially use the patient as a database to determine what information is already mastered. You then "fill in the void" with the correct amount of information which you think is important for a particular patient.

Determining the last four elements: patient's ability to learn, and the method of instruction, time of instruction, and evaluation of learning are difficult and require training which goes beyond the scope of this chapter. You are referred to the work by Bernstein and Bernstein in the references. The remaining sections of this chapter will focus on the first three components of the educational diagnosis and patient interviewing skills.

The process of interviewing goes beyond asking a series of pre-planned questions in a certain order. Although this approach may be effective in some aspects of pharmacy care, such as screening for hypertension, it may not be the most appropriate approach in other situations, such as when patients are reluctant to talk about their problems (Bernstein, et al., 1980). The basic skills discussed in this unit can be used in a variety of settings or situations, and, if used properly, can greatly enhance the efficiency of the interview and the quality of information provided.

COMPONENTS OF AN EFFECTIVE INTERVIEW

As mentioned earlier, conducting an effective interview is not a simple process. The interview process contains several critical components that need to be mastered. The process is somewhat analogous to learning to drive a car. At first, you must learn specific skills, such as using the clutch, applying the brakes properly, and using the rearview mirror. Once these skills have been learned, the process becomes automatic and rather simple — until you have an accident. Then you must analyze what went wrong with your skills (e.g., you didn't use the turn signal, or you miscalculated your speed on a curve); the driving skill is then corrected or relearned, and you continue on safely. The same is true with effective interviewing. Certain communication and interviewing skills need to be mastered and used or you might have an "accident" or an unproductive interview. The accident can be minor (e.g., you miss one piece of information) or major (e.g., the patient stomps out of the pharmacy vowing never to return). By considering the elements of effective interviewing in this chapter you will be able to avoid accidents and analyze what went wrong if one does occur.

Listening

In general, people are better senders of information than receivers of information. We have been taught how to improve our verbal and written communication skills, but not our listening skills. Thus, we must concentrate much harder on the listening component of the communication process. Nothing will end an interview faster than having patients realize that you are not listening to them. Although listening skills have been discussed in Chapter 5, the following recommendations relating to interviewing specifically are addressed below:

1. Stop talking. You can't listen while you are talking.

2. Get rid of distractions. These break your concentration.

3. Use good eye contact (i.e., look at the other person). This helps you concentrate and shows the other person that you are indeed listening.

4. React to ideas, not to the person. Focus on what is being said and not on whether you like the person.

5. Read nonverbal messages. These may communicate the same or a different message than the one given verbally.

6. Listen to how something is said. The tone of voice and rate of speech also transmit part of the message.

7. Provide feedback to clarify any messages. This also shows that you are listening and trying to understand.

Probing

Another important communication skill is learning to ask questions in a way that elicits the most accurate information. This technique is called "probing." Probing is the use of questions to elicit needed information from patients or to help clarify their problems. Asking questions seems to be a straightforward task, which it is in most situations. However, several things should be considered before asking a question. The phrasing of the question is important. Patients are often put on the defensive by questions that seem to put them ill at ease. For instance, "why" type questions should be avoided, because they make people feel they have to justify why they did a certain thing. It is better to use "what" or "how" type of questions. For example, many people might be defensive if asked "Why are you taking these medications?" instead of "For what reasons are you taking this medication?"

In addition, timing of the question is important. Several questions in succession may leave the patient with a sense of being interrogated and therefore may raise her level of defensiveness. The patient should be allowed to finish answering the current question before proceeding on to the next one. If you must obtain information quickly, prepare the patient by using a warning such as "I know this might seem rude, but in order to get the needed information I have to ask you quite a few questions in the next few minutes." Also, leading questions should be avoided. These questions strongly imply an expected answer (for example, "You usually don't forget to take the medication, do you?"). These questions lead the patient into discussing what she thinks you want to hear rather than what the patient needs to tell you. Exceptions to this principle occur when you want to explore a specific area. Carefully phrased leading questions can bring out into the open problems not easily discussed. For example, "When did you first begin to feel depressed?"

To conduct an effective interview, it is important to understand the differences between closed-ended and open-ended questions. A closed-ended question can be answered with either a "yes" or "no" response or with a few words at most. On the other hand, an open-ended question neither limits the patient's response nor induces defensiveness. For example, a closed-ended question would be "Has your doctor told you how to take this medication?" The patient may only respond with a "yes" or "no" and not provide any useful information to you. An example of an open-ended question would be "How has your doctor told you to take this medication?" The phrasing of this question allows the patient to state exactly how she perceives the medication should be taken. Proper open-ended questions are harder to formulate than closed-ended questions, but they are more crucial in decreasing the patient's defensiveness by conveying a willingness on your part to listen. With an open-ended question you are allowing patients to present their own points of view.

Closed-ended questions reduce the patient's degree of openness and cause the patient to become more passive during the interviewing process because you are doing most of the talking. Closed-ended questions also enable patients to avoid specific subjects and emotional expression. Closed-ended questions can connote an air of interrogation and impersonality. For this reason closed-ended questions are referred to as "pharmacist-centered questions." Open-ended questions do not require the other person to respond in your frame of reference. Open-ended questions permit open expression and for this reason are sometimes referred to as "patient-centered questions." Closed-ended questions are necessary and are indeed useful; however, open-ended questions are less likely to result in misunderstanding, and they tend to promote rapport and develop trusting relationships.

You may find a combination of open-ended and closed-ended questions most efficient for you in your practice. Patient encounters may be initiated with an open-ended question, followed by more directed, closed-ended questions. For example, if you want to know if Mr. Raymond is experiencing bothersome side effects from his antihypertensive medication, you may say, "How have you been feeling?" and/or "What brings you into the clinic today?" If necessary, these questions can be followed with: "What type of things have you noticed after taking this medication?" If necessary, this question can be followed by: "How bothersome are these side effects?" If necessary, this question can then be followed by more direct questioning: "Have you been awakened during the night?" "Do you have trouble sleeping?" "Do you feel weak?" "Do you feel tired?" and so on.

Interviews comprised principally of closed-ended questions make you the problem solver rather than the facilitator of problem solving — that is, asking questions implies that you will come up with answers. Experience has found that open-ended questions are more effective in assessing patient understanding as seen in the "educational diagnosis" sequence. The Indian Health Service has developed an effective patient education program which uses a series of open-ended questions during the patient assessment process (see Gardner, et al., 1991).

In summary, be aware of when and how you ask a question. The ultimate test is this: will the question I am about to ask be helpful to the other person? When a question is needed, open-ended questions elicit more complete and unabridged information that does not squeeze the patient into your perspective. Open-ended questions convey a willingness to listen. Conversely, closed-ended questions reduce openness and encourage passivity and avoidance of specifics and emotional expression. Open-ended questions are almost always better than closed-ended questions because they yield more information. Of course, in some situations a simple "yes" or "no" answer will be necessary. It takes practice to develop a good questioning technique that uses a combination of both closed- and open-ended questions to move the interview to its conclusion. Tact must be developed when you use open-ended questions to prevent patients from wandering off into subject areas that might not be relevant to the situation.

Use of Silence

Another skill that you must learn is the art of using silence appropriately. During the interview, there will be times when neither you nor the patient will speak, especially in the early moments. You must learn to treat these pauses as a necessary part of the process and not be uncomfortable with them. Many times, the patient needs time to think or react to the information you have provided. Interrupting the silence destroys the opportunity for the patient to think about this material. On the other hand, the pause might be due to the fact that the patient did not understand the question completely. In this situation, the question should be restated or rephrased. At the same time, too much silence when the patient is expressing feelings such as fear or depression may be interpreted as rejection by you. The patient may be looking for some type of response from you.

In any event, you should avoid the temptation to fill empty spaces in the interview with unnecessary talk. In fact, some studies have found that the more the "talk ratio" is in favor of the interviewee, the more likely that the interview will be successful. Thus, the patient should be able to relax and be allowed time to think during the necessary pauses in the interview process.

Establishing Rapport

Successful interviews are marked by a high degree of rapport between the two parties. Rapport is built mainly on mutual consideration and respect. It is difficult to achieve rapport in some cases, because it is a two-way process. You can aid this process by using a sincere, friendly greeting, by being courteous during the discussion, and by not stereotyping or prejudging the patient. Each patient must be seen as a unique individual. The ability to establish rapport is enhanced when patients use the same pharmacy for their pharmacy services. So, when first meeting a patient urge them to only use one pharmacy.

INTERVIEWING AS A PROCESS

Proper planning and sequencing of the interview are essential in carrying out an effective patient assessment. Before an interview is started, several decisions must be made regarding how it will be conducted. The type of approach usually depends on the type of information desired and the environment available for it.

Type of Information

Before the interview begins, you should determine the amount and type of information desired. In other words, what exactly do you want to accomplish? For example, if you need to find out specific pieces of information, you need to have more control over the interview process. This is referred to as the directed interview approach. However, if the outcome is unknown or somewhat ambiguous, you need to use the nondirected approach. This approach allows the interview to become more free flowing; the points of discussion are raised by the patient rather than by you. When you use this approach, you hope the problem or concern will surface, allowing you to deal with it. In the nondirected approach, open-ended questions should be used more frequently than closed-ended questions. However, even in the directed approach you can ask an initial open-ended question to assess their understanding as discussed earlier.

Type of Environment

Planning for the interview must include consideration of the type of environment available. The environment is critical, because one of the fundamental principles of interviewing is to provide as much privacy as possible. Research has shown that the degree of privacy is related to many critical outcomes of the interview process (for example, the level of patient understanding of the medication and the degree of compliance with the treatment regimen). As the privacy of the setting improves, the amount of information retained by the patient increases, along with the likelihood that the patient will take the prescribed medication correctly. Privacy also allows both you and the patient to express personal concerns, to ask difficult questions, to listen more effectively, and to share honest opinions. Unfortunately, the setting of the interview in many pharmacies — over a busy prescription counter or in other areas where distractions abound — is not always the best. Before you begin the interview, interruptions should be reduced as much as possible. A partition at the end of the prescription counter, a special room, or a consulting area can provide the necessary privacy.

Starting the Interview

After considering the type of environment available and the type of information desired, you should start the interview by greeting the patient sincerely and by introducing yourself to the patient if you do not know her. This helps establish rapport with the patient. You should also state the purpose of the interview, outline what will happen during the interview, and put the patient at ease. The amount of time needed, the subjects to be covered, and the final outcome should be mentioned so that the patient has a clear understanding of the process. For example, a pharmacist seeing a patient for the first time might say:

> "Hi, I'm Jane Bradley, the pharmacist (the introduction), and I would like to ask you a few quick questions about the drugs you are now taking (the subjects to be covered). This will take only a few minutes (the amount of time needed) and will allow me to create a drug profile so that I can keep track of all the medications that you are taking. This will help us identify potential problems with new medications you might be prescribed (the purpose/outcome)."

Such a beginning allows you to define the limits and expectations of the interview so that the patient remains comfortable and does not have other expectations about the interview. After the interview is started, the following suggestions will help you conduct a more efficient interview:

1. Avoid making recommendations during the information-gathering phases of the interview. Such recommendations prevent the patient from giving you all the needed information.

2. Similarly, do not jump to conclusions or rapid solutions without hearing all the facts.

3. Do not shift from one subject to another until it the first has been followed through.

4. Guide the interview using a combination of open- and closed-ended questions.

5. Similarly, keep your goals clearly in mind, but do not let them dominate how you go about the interview.

6. Maintain objectivity by not allowing the patient's attitudes, beliefs, or prejudices to influence your thinking.

7. Use good communication skills, especially the probing, listening, and feedback components.

8. Be aware of the patient's nonverbal messages, because these signal how the interview is progressing.

9. Depending on your relationship with the patient, move from general to more specific questions, and less personal to more personal subjects. This may remove some of the patient's initial defensiveness.

10. Note-taking should be as brief as possible, because lengthy entries tend to create suspicion.

Ending the Interview

Bringing the interview to a close is often more difficult than starting the interview. It is a crucial part of the interview process because a person's evaluation of the entire interview and your performance may be based on the final statements. People seem to remember best what was said last. Therefore, care should be taken not to end the interview abruptly or to rush the patient out the door.

To conclude the interview, a short summary may be necessary. A summary allows both parties the opportunity to review exactly what has been discussed and helps clarify any misunderstanding. It is essential that both people agree about what has been said. A summary provides a time for you to ask the patient to repeat key information (provide feedback) back to you so that you can reinforce important points and correct any misinformation. A summary also sets the stage for future patient contact and expectations that you both have of one another. A summary also tactfully hints to the patient that the interview is ending. In conjunction with a summary you can use nonverbal cues to indicate to the patient that the interview is over. For instance, you could get up from the chair or change your stance in such a way that indicates that you need to move on. A simple closed-ended question such as "Do you have any further questions?" or a sincere statement such as "I enjoyed talking to you. If you think of something you forgot to mention or have questions when you get home, please give me a call" may also be useful. The ending of the interview is a good time for you to reassure the patient about a particular problem. However, this should not be false assurance, such as "Everything is going to turn out okay" or "Don't worry about it." Instead, you should state, "I (or we) will try to help things get better for you." Finally, before terminating the interaction, you should reflect on whether the goals of the interview were accomplished (final step in the educational diagnosis process) and what should be done if they were not.

INTERVIEWING USING THE TELEPHONE

Many times you need to collect information from patients by telephone. In light of the importance of the telephone, you should strive to maximize its effective use. Effective telephone skills can also help create a positive image for your pharmacy and lend support to your professional credibility. In addition, proficient telephone communication can contribute to personnel productivity and, ultimately, to the professional and financial success of your pharmacy. The following should be considered during this type of interaction:

1.   Cue yourself to smile before you pick up the telephone. Your friendly attitude will be transmitted through the tone, pitch, volume, and inflection of your voice.

2.   If at all possible, answer the telephone or have a fellow employee answer it within the first three or four rings.

3.   Identify the pharmacy and yourself, providing both your name and position. (e.g., Professional Pharmacy, Jane Jones speaking. May I help you?") While it may appear burdensome to identify yourself fully to every caller, you should keep in mind that each call may represent the first contact the caller has with you and your pharmacy. Even if it is not the first contact, each call is a uniquely important communication for the caller and should be given your full attention.

4. Give your full attention to the call. Perhaps nothing is more irritating to a caller than to be given the impression that she is competing for your attention.

5. Ask for the caller's name and use her name in the conversation, particularly at the conclusion of the call. Not only does this reduce possible confusion and error, but by asking for and using the caller's name, you project a more personal, empathic attitude.

6. If you must place the caller on hold, or simply leave the telephone (for a short time only), ask, "May I put you on hold while I look up your prescription?" In these circumstances, it is important that you do the following:

    a. tell the caller why you want to put them on hold;

    b. ask if she would mind waiting a brief time, or would prefer to call back (if appropriate); and,

    c. on returning to the telephone, say, "Thank you for waiting."

7. At the conclusion of the call, end it graciously (e.g., "Thank you for calling"). Do not, however, overdo your graciousness. Lines such as "Thank you ever so much for doing business with us" will only convey insincerity.

8. Finally, if possible allow the caller to hang up first. This will allow her time to remember that extra request. It will also project in a subtle manner your sincere desire to listen.

Besides receiving telephone calls, many times you must call physicians or other health care professionals to obtain additional information regarding a patient. The following suggestions may help make these calls more efficient.

1. Before you pick up the receiver, be sure you have any and all information related to the call readily available. Prescription, patient, and other relevant information should be obtained before your telephone conversation starts.

2. Before you pick up the receiver, determine whom you need to speak with to achieve your purpose for calling.

3. Most importantly, before you pick up the receiver ask yourself, "Is this call necessary?"

4. Identify yourself, your position, and the pharmacy first. Then ask (if it is not already provided to you) for the same information from the person who has answered your call.

5. Immediately after introducing yourself, state in clear, concise terms the reason for your call. Be assertive! Do not begin by apologizing ("Sorry to bother you"). You have already decided that the call is necessary.

6. If the nature of your call dictates that it will exceed more than a couple of minutes, ask the person if they have time to talk with you for a few minutes.

7. Conclude the conversation with a sincere "Thank you."

SUMMARY

Conducting patient assessment is a complex process that at times is difficult to master, because it involves interactions between two persons. No two interactions are exactly the same, because the sequence of events and the people involved are never exactly the same. Interviews require different levels of flexibility based on the needs of the patient; they also require some type of structure to assure a timely, clear transmission of information between you and the patient. In order to conduct a successful interview, certain communication skills need to be mastered. If the two parties are not communicating well, the entire interview process can break down, and the possibility of future positive interactions between the patient and pharmacist can be jeopardized. You must learn how to ask open-ended questions, to transmit information clearly, listen effectively, provide feedback, use silence, and develop rapport. Development of these skills takes time. In addition to using good communication skills, you must realize how to structure the interview. The type of environment, the type of approach, and how to start and how to end the interview are all critical to the interview process.

The first step in improving this process is to realize that the effective use of these skills will lead to a more productive interview. You should evaluate each interview by asking such questions as "Did the patient appear to be relaxed and open?" or "Did I check to see if the patient knew what I was talking about?" Such an analysis will reveal some interesting things and will point to possible areas of improvement.

The interview is a dynamic process that can always be improved. You cannot rest on previous successes, because many things in the process can be improved. At the same time, you should not worry about saying the wrong thing or putting your foot in your mouth. After making a blunder, people have a tendency to shy away from further interactions with other patients. Experience has shown that most patients are forgiving; and relationships can be salvaged after a negative encounter. The key is to identify what went wrong, correct it, and move on to the next interview.

REFERENCES

Bernstein L, and Bernstein RS: *Interviewing: A Guide for Health Professionals.* New York: Appleton-Century-Crofts, 1980.

Gardner MG, Boyce RW, Herrier RN: *Pharmacist-patient Consultation Program: An Interactive Approach to Verify Patient Understanding.* New York: Pfizer-Roerig, 1991.

RECOMMENDED READINGS

Beardsley RS, Johnson CA, and Wise G: Privacy as a factor in patient counseling. J. Am. Pharm. Assoc., *NS17:*366, 1977.

Covington T, and Whitney HAK Jr: Patient-pharmacist communication techniques. Drug Intell. Clin. Pharm., *5:*370, 1971.

Ivey PW, and Manolis M: Patient-pharmacist interview. Drug Intell. Clin. Pharm., *32:*828, 1975.

Keys PW, and Manolis M: Patient-pharmacist interview. Drug Intell. Clin. Pharm., *12:*400, 1978.

Lawrence D: If I were in his shoes, how would I feel? J. Am. Pharm. Assoc., *NS16:*453, 1976.

Storrow JA: *Outline of Clinical Psychiatry.* New York: Appleton-Century-Crofts, 1969.

CHAPTER 8

How to Build Better Patient Understanding

OVERVIEW

This chapter presents techniques to build better patient understanding. Such understanding is essential in helping patients meet therapeutic goals. It presupposes that the patient-pharmacist dialogue is focused on meeting patients' needs; that these needs can be assessed through open-ended questions; and that meeting these needs will improve patients' understanding of their medication and their overall therapy.

INTRODUCTION

An ancient physician once approached his colleagues with this admonition: "Keep watch also on the fault of patients which often makes them lie about taking of things prescribed." It appears that when Hippocrates made this remark he had already observed noncompliant behavior over 2,000 years ago. More recently another physician, Frank E. Young, M.D., Ph.D., a former Commissioner of the United States Food and Drug Administration (FDA), added his observation to this millennia-old problem by stating: "The basic and most common cause of noncompliance is the patient who does not understand what is expected." The current (1993) FDA Commissioner, David Kessler, M.D., has stated, "Evidence suggests that inadequate communication about drugs is one of the principal reasons why 30-55% of patients deviate from their medication regimens" (Kessler, D.A., 1991). Up to this point, several elements in the communication process have been emphasized, i.e., empathy, respect, and warmth. These elements facilitate communication because they encourage the pharmacist and the patient to explore feelings about the patient's health as well as to examine medication use and any associated problems. This exploration will reveal problems the patient may have and facilitate the development of a professional relationship focused on enhancing teamwork and mutual accountability.

During the last twenty-five years, an increasing body of literature on the patient's role in medical care often cites a conflict between the patient's need for autonomy and the values of the patient's care givers (Emanuel, 1992). Preferring to diminish the professional's role in favor of patient autonomy, some literature advocates more patient control in health decisions (Macklin, 1987) or a more mutually accountable relationship (Marzuk, 1985). This second argument is defended on the basis that, at times, the patient's reasoning may be in a diminished state or the patient may need a health professional to help him understand highly technical medical situations, jargon, and treatment protocols (Siegler, 1985). In addition, because as many as 85% of patients are reluctant to ask questions about their health or drugs, pharmacists must not be reluctant to initiate conversations to help them understand their medication. As one practitioner has put it, "Patients are usually shy" (White, 1991).

PHARMACISTS' RELUCTANCE TO ASSESS UNDERSTANDING

Pharmacists usually know what to tell patients about their medicines, but for many reasons, they view the process as a one-way communication. Their practice behavior may simply be to talk *to* the patient, and thus they fail to ask for feedback necessary to identify a patient's lack of understanding about their medication.

A useful first step in improving patient counseling would be for a pharmacist to first identify any of his own beliefs or behaviors that influence and hinder his communication effectiveness (Leibowitz, 1993). A second step would be for the pharmacist to examine his attitude toward medications. Pharmacists often see their central and most important role as "dispensing," and with that infer that the patient will also view obtaining the medication as important and valued. The pharmacist may rationalize, "This medication must be important to the patient or else why did he patronize my pharmacy, pay $65.00 for it, wait a half hour for it, and then ask five questions about it?"

Pharmacists may forget that obtaining any prescription and initiating any medication regimen involves an interruption in the patient's everyday priorities of life, e.g., working, shopping, chauffeuring the children, getting the laundry done, preparing dinner, attending a PTA meeting, and so on. Some pharmacists tend to believe that if they tell a patient about a medication regimen, then because they have "told them" it becomes an important priority around which the patient's life will soon revolve. In reality, most people do lead more or less organized, habitual, or patterned lives, and the taking of medications becomes an interruption to that order that is difficult to integrate unless something else gives way.

If improved understanding is a goal of patient counseling, then to accomplish it, pharmacists will have to view patients as busy, absorbed, distracted, distraught, and engaged in a variety of activities and relationships. Their visit to a pharmacist is just one more of life's events to cope with. To protect patients from the limitations of a diminished understanding about their medicine, pharmacists must perceive the patient as a whole being. Desired medication outcomes can be best achieved if a caring, trusting relationship between pharmacist and patient can be built on some base of mutual respect and accountability.

A third reason for some pharmacists' lack of initiating patient conversation is that they have assimilated their helping model based upon the traditions of the medical model. In medicine, "helping" was originally viewed as a process of (1) gathering information about the patient, (2) diagnosing the patient's condition, and (3) prescribing a treatment for that condition. As pharmacy evolved into a more clinical role, this same process was modified so that pharmacists (1) gather information about the patient, (2) consult with the prescriber, and (3) collaborate in the treatment plan. One problem with such a model is that it develops a thinking pattern that places too much emphasis on "What is the process that I, the professional, must follow?" vs. "What is it that this patient truly needs?" It becomes too easy for health professionals to "understand" noncompliant behavior by labeling the patient as: neurotic, depressed, resistant, suffering side effects, having an "attitude," or some other conclusion that leaves the professional blameless. This easy way of casting the patient into a negative light gets the pharmacist "off the hook." Pharmacists can rationalize themselves as being blameless for not helping the patient understand what was expected relative to medication use. Changing the professional's viewpoint of his responsibilities can cause him to communicate differently. For example, instead of offering a "stereotyped" patient a standardized response, pharmacists can individualize their patient encounters by asking questions that assess a patient's understanding. The remaining counseling time can be used to fill in information gaps or offer suggestions that improve compliant behavior. For example, a pharmacist may suggest to the patient who is living alone, and who is more likely to have compliance problems, to enlist a neighbor or coworker for help in following a medication regimen.

Pharmacists must also keep in mind that there is an imperfect tie between taking medications as prescribed and reaching desired therapeutic outcomes. Patients may alter the dose of a drug and still have blood levels within therapeutic range or be "controlled" symptomatically. Thus, before intervening to improve compliance, pharmacists must first assess exactly what the effects of the patient's current medication-taking practices have been on medical outcomes. In all cases, the goal of a pharmacist's intervention is *not* to get patients to do as they are told (e.g. comply) — the goal instead is to help the patient reach desired medical and quality-of-life outcomes. Compliance with drug therapy is often a means to help reach the goal but it is not a goal in itself.

The pharmacist's challenge is to help motivate the patient (Lasagna, 1992) into staying with a treatment regimen when the harm for not doing so may not be readily apparent to the patient. Noncompliance is particularly problematic among those on chronic medications such as antihypertensives where patients cannot perceive improvements in how they feel that are closely tied to medication use.

Research (McKenney, et al., 1978) shows that the quality of communication between patient and health care providers, if friendly and positive, will improve understanding and ultimately lead to better compliance. In addition, patient satisfaction with their health professional is related to how well patients adhere to treatment regimens (McKenney, et al., 1978; Smith, et al., 1981). Some studies also indicate that certain noncompliance is due to economic factors. For example, unemployed or elderly patients (Cooper, et al., 1982) may decide to take every other tablet in order to "stretch" limited resources. Other patients may be subject to work-related stress and become so preoccupied that they cannot focus on their need to take medication at prescribed times, especially bedtime doses. Thus, caring pharmacists, by considering all these factors, can rethink their professional responsibilities and do much to help meet patient needs.

Communication to achieve better understanding is often complex. Many people find sharing private matters difficult and therefore they resist developing a relationship in which teamwork is the goal. If patients feel there is no rapport between them and their pharmacist, two-way communication will be diminished and ultimately patient care will suffer.

FALSE ASSUMPTIONS ABOUT PATIENT UNDER-STANDING

Pharmacists are in a strong position to help patients avoid medication-related problems. But to do this they must have a clear picture of what medications a patient takes, how he takes them, problems he perceives with medication use, and other information. This means asking the right questions and empathically listening to the answers. Pharmacists should not assume, or take for granted, that they know the answers to questions they have not asked. Some of the following assumptions must be kept in mind, as these interfere with a pharmacist's ability to understand patients' medication use.

1. Do not assume that physicians have already discussed with patients the medications they prescribe. In fact, one study shows that physicians frequently omit critical information (Svarstad, 1986). This study found that with 17% of the prescriptions written by physicians during office visits, no explicit directions for use were given. Clear instructions on duration of use were given only 10% of the time, and instructions for frequency of use were given only 17% of the time.

2. Do not assume that patients understand all information given. Research has indicated that even seemingly straightforward label directions like "take one (1) tablet every six (6) hours" can be interpreted by a large percentage of patients to mean three doses during a waking day.

3. Do not assume that, if patients understand what is required, they have all the tools necessary to comply. Implementing a new medication regimen requires a change in behavior,

which can be difficult. Anyone who has tried to change old habits or implement new ones — a new diet or exercise regimen for example — knows how hard that can be. Pharmacists should be able to promote a patient's "self-efficacy" (Cameron, 1987). This will require that the pharmacist know something about the patient's life-style as well as work, personal, and professional atmosphere, support and coping mechanisms (Ell, 1986), and then fold that knowledge into his counseling interventions.

4. Do not assume when communication breaks down that the patient "doesn't care," "isn't motivated," "lacks intelligence," or "can't remember" (especially the elderly). These assumptions prevent pharmacists from taking a full partnering role in helping patients manage their own drug therapy. The professional literature has yet to yield research that establishes a relationship between personal characteristics and adherence to medical advice. It does, however, show that achievement of desired outcomes is related to the degree to which patient-provider communication is effective (Hill, 1989). Depending on the study, estimates are that 35–92% of patients do not understand information given to them, and about 40% of the information that is provided is soon forgotten (Ley, 1985). On the other hand, if comprehension, memory, and satisfaction are increased modestly, compliance rates could be improved dramatically (Ley, 1985).

5. Do not assume that once a patient understands how to comply with a medication regimen, compliant behavior will occur. Evidence suggests that pharmacists should reinforce their patient counseling and drug monitoring on a regular basis. Once this reinforcement stops, patients often slip into noncompliant behavior.

6. Do not assume that physicians routinely monitor their patients' use of medications and, if there are medication problems, that the prescriber knows them and is addressing them. Careful drug monitoring and its related clinical assessments are activities frequently missing from the pharmacist-physician-patient relationship.

7. Do not assume that, if patients are having problems, they will ask direct questions or volunteer information. A pharmacist with this mindset will erroneously assume that all he has to do is be willing to address problems raised by the patient so that the burden of starting communications is removed from the pharmacist. This assumption ignores the fact that patients may misunderstand the regimen or may be embarrassed to admit having problems. The pharmacist must take responsibility as an initiator, an investigator into problems, and, most of all, a problem solver who seeks to help patients overcome barriers to appropriate medication use by helping patients build a complete understanding of their medication therapy.

TECHNIQUES TO ASSESS PATIENT UNDERSTANDING

To best help patients, pharmacists need information about a patient's beliefs, understandings, and actual medication use. To do this they must begin by asking the patient questions. Chapter 7 focused on effective interviewing. This chapter now builds on that information by making suggestions on how to assess a patient's understanding and medication use so that counseling interventions might be made.

Assessing Patient Understanding of Medication

Since patients must understand what is expected of them so that they can take their medications appropriately, pharmacists should find out what patient understanding is being brought to the conversation. This could prevent the pharmacist from offering already understood information or poorly understood jargon which wastes time. Time can then be devoted to filling in gaps or correcting misconceptions. Here are some open-ended questions that help assess what a patient understands because they prompt detailed responses and encourage a more complete disclosure of information.

1. What did your doctor tell you about this medicine?

2. How did your doctor tell you to take the medicine?

3. What exactly is your medicine supposed to do?

4. What medical problem has caused you to need this medicine?

5. What special instructions or precautions were you given?

Assessing Understanding of Medication Use

Some questions for you to ask are:

1. At what times during the day do you plan to take your medicine?

2. Will these times be convenient for you?

3. How should you be storing this medicine?

Assessing Potential Problems with Medication Use

In assessing possible reasons for non-compliance itself, you might ask:

1. If you ever skip doses or forget to take your medicine, why do you think this happens?

2. What did your doctor tell you to do if you missed a dose?

3. When, if ever, did you forget your medication this past week?

4. How long are you going to be taking this medicine?

Assessing Other Medication Problems

The pharmacist then uses open-ended questioning to help the patient identify other problems, such as adverse drug reactions and inability to afford the medications. Questions might include:

1. What side effects, if any, have you experienced since you started taking this medicine?

2. What effects are you supposed to watch out for?

3. How will you know if your medication is working?

4. What will you do if your medicine doesn't seem to work?

Assessing Other Health Problems

Pharmacists need to be sure to assess what other Rx and OTC medications patients may be taking, as well as how they perceive the medicine they are about to take. As perceptions affect compliance behavior and misperceptions can be barriers to it, the pharmacist who identifies problems can make suggestions regarding the importance of and reasons for following instructions as a way to correct misperceptions or reinforce correct perceptions. Such questions might include:

1. What non-prescription medicine might you be taking?

2. How well does your medication seem to be working?

3. Do you have any problems in taking this medication that we haven't discussed?

4. How do you feel about having to take this expensive medication (if cost is a possible barrier)?

5. What do you think will happen to your health if you don't take the medicine as prescribed?

Note that the authors are suggesting that the pharmacist do more than simply tell a patient about their medication. A telling approach may leave out over half of the communication process, i.e., the acquisition of feedback that allows one to know a message is understood. Thus, there is a need for pharmacists to apply the simple technique of using open-ended questions that begin with the use of who, how, when, where, what, and why during patient counseling. These questions induce the patient to give more than a "yes or no" response and encourage the patient to provide information which the pharmacist can use to assess the patient's understanding of a particular situation. As the patient encounter continues, the pharmacist can then use assessment of the patient's understanding to fill in gaps of knowledge or reinforce salient points. When gathering information with open-ended questions, the pharmacist can occasionally control and direct the conversation by using more focused and specific questioning. Pharmacists would do well to remember that effective communication (see Table 1, Epilogue) requires one to verify the meaning of a message and to accept the feelings and perceptions of others.

TECHNIQUES TO IMPROVE PATIENT UNDERSTANDING

Once a pharmacist has assessed a patient's understanding of his/ medication, the pharmacist can help patients comply with treatment regimens by filling in the information gaps with easy-to-understand language. Suggested behavior management techniques that facilitate compliance and improve the efficacy of the patient counseling encounter are expanded below and are referenced in the epilogue (Table 2, Epilogue). Pharmacists need only look at the world around them to see how these practical, proven techniques are being used to change other social behaviors such as wearing seat belts, recycling glass and newspaper, exercising, reducing cholesterol intake, and most of all, stopping smoking.

1. Emphasize key points. Telling a patient beforehand, "Now this is very important" helps him remember what follows.

2. Give reasons for key advice. Tell why it is necessary to continue using an antibiotic even though symptoms have disap-

peared. Information well understood is information more easily remembered and more likely to be followed.

3. Give definite, concrete, explicit instructions. Any information we can mentally picture is more easily remembered. Use visual aids, photographs, or demonstrations. When patients are given specific, easy-to-understand instructions, they tend to regard this advice as more important than that which is given in general terms.

4. Supplement and reinforce the spoken word with written instructions. By so doing, you can pare face-to-face consultations down to essentials and, at the same time, provide your patient with information to refer to as needed.

5. Finally, no communication encounter, especially one designed to be helpful, should end without the kind of feedback that lets both patient and pharmacist understand the salient points of the encounter. Thus, before a pharmacist lets a patient leave, he should ask the patient to restate one or two critical points in order to check for accuracy. At this point, the pharmacist should assume accountability for the adequacy of his consultation by a statement such as: "I'd appreciate another moment of your time in which I'd like you to tell me just when exactly you're going to take this medication" or "I want to be sure I didn't leave anything out, so you would you please state what your dosing schedule will be and how you're going to store this."

The use of these open-ended questions to assess a patient's understanding, then filling in gaps or adding salient information, is a process that does enhance the OBRA '90 requirements for patient counseling. In fact, it makes the accepted offer of counseling an interactive affair resulting in an efficient, effective use of time. For example, if a patient can tell a pharmacist he knows the drug's name, storage issues, dosing schedule, and a few common side effects, then the pharmacist need only introduce pertinent, missing points or briefly reinforce that which is already understood.

CHANGING BEHAVIOR AFTER CHANGING UNDERSTANDING

Once a pharmacist has honed his patient communication skills and has assimilated the techniques of an effective counseling session, then he can focus on various behavior management techniques that will help with medication compliance (see Table 3 in Epilogue):

1. It is hard for someone to establish a new behavior unless it is tied to an existing behavior. Thus, pharmacists can help patients name events in daily routines that can be tied to taking medication. If such habits do not exist, then patients can be helped to find other reminders. For example, a prescription says, "Take three (3) times a day with meals." If that patient does not eat lunch, a midday dose may be missed. If the patient cannot identify a reminder event, suggest the setting of a wristwatch or other alarm, or posting reminder notes in an obvious place, or storing the medication where it will be seen at the time it is due to be taken.

2. Suggest ways to self-monitor. One simple way to help patients is the suggestion that they use a medication diary or calendar on which to record their medication use. Individualized medication packaging for daily or weekly doses are also available suggestions. Patients who use such devices can tell when a dose is due and whether or not they have already taken it. Digital time pieces are commonplace today and are installed in some vial caps. They sound an alarm for the next dose or measure the time since the last dose. Patients can also be taught to monitor their own responses to treatment. For example, teaching patients how to take their own blood pressure readings can be a strong reinforcement regarding their medication use. For example, the pharmacist could state: "Now that we both understand how you will be taking your medicine and you understand how important it is to keep your blood pressure down, would you like me to show you how you can take your own blood pressure?"

3.   Monitor compliance. With chronic care medications, you should frequently monitor compliance as well as patient perceptions of effectiveness and problems encountered. Review profile records for indications of problems, such as patterns of late refills. Refill-reminder software systems are available to help. Call patients to see how they are doing after they start on a new prescription. Assess compliance and problems in follow-up visits. Maintain periodic monitoring even if your patient seems to have no problems initially. Research shows that patient compliance frequently stops when the pharmacist's attention stops.

4.   In some cases, pharmacists' response may require referring patients to a social service agency or government program that can help, such as one for low-income patients. A call to a county information-and-referral number should put them in touch with local resources. In any case, it requires actively listening to the patients' perceptions of treatment. Dismissing patient concerns will not make their problems go away. It may, more often than not, result in patients who fail to comply and then hide their noncompliance from a health care professional who could have helped them get the best outcomes from their medications if they had been better aware of patient needs.

SUMMARY

Assessment of patient understanding as part of the patient counseling process is a fragile system that can be rendered ineffective by a pharmacist's misperceptions about the patient and assumptions about the practice of taking prescribed medication. To help patients become more self-directed at taking their medication, pharmacists first must develop a feedback system that lets *them* understand what patients understand about their medications. Only then can they assess the causes and effects of noncompliant behavior and make suggestions to improve therapeutic outcomes. Techniques to improve patient communication in a counseling encounter, which in turn leads to a better use of medications, can be learned easily and do make a difference to the quality of life of both pharmacist and patient.

REFERENCES

Cameron R: Promoting adherence to health behavior. Patient Educ. Counsel, *10*:139-54, 1987.

Cooper JK, et al.: Intentional prescription nonadherence by the elderly. J. of Am. Geriatrics Society, *5*:329-33, 1982.

Ell KO: Coping with serious illness. Int. J. Psychiatric Med., *15*:335-56, 1986.

Emanuel EJ, et al.: Tour models of the physician patient relationship. JAMA, *267*(16), 2221-26, April 22, 1992.

Hill MN: Strategies for patient education. Clinical and Experimental Hypertension, *A11*:5-6, 1989.

Kessler DA: Communicating with patients about their medicine. NEJM, *325*(23), Dec. 1991.

Lasagna L: Noncompliance data and clinical outcomes. Drug Topics Supplement *136*(10), 1992.

Leibowitz K: Improving your patient counseling skills. Am. Pharmacy, *N533*(4): 65-69, April 1993.

Ley P: Doctor-patient relationships. J. of Hypertension, *3*: 51-55, 1985.

Macklin R: *Mortal Choices*. New York: Pantheon Books, 1987.

Marzuk PM: The right kind of paternalism. New England Journal of Medicine, *313*:1474-76, 1985.

McKenney JM, Brown ED, Necsary R, and Reavis HL: Effect of pharmacist drug monitoring and patient education on hypertensive patients. Contemporary Pharmacy Practice, *1*:50-56, 1978.

Siegler M: The progression of medicine. Arch. Intern. Med., *145*:713-715, 1985.

Smith C, Polis E, and Hadac R: Characteristics of the initial medical interview associated with patient satisfaction and understanding. J. Fam. Pract., *12*:283-288, 1981.

Svarstad BL: Patient-practitioner relationships and compliance with prescribed medical regimens. In Aiken LH, ed.: *Applic. of Social Sciences to Clinical Medicine on Health Policy*. New Brunswick, NJ: Rutgers University Press, pp. 438-459, 1986.

White SJ, et al.: Patient education: How practitioners see it. Am. Pharmacy, *NS231*(7):402-02, 1991.

RECOMMENDED READING

Becker MH, and Maiman LA: Sociobehavioral determinants of compliance with health and medical care recommendations. Medical Care, *13*(1):10-24, 1975.

DiMatteo MR, Hays RD, and Prince LM: Relationship of physicians' nonverbal communication skill to patient satisfaction, appointment noncompliance, and physician workload. Health Psychology, *5*:581-594, 1986.

Freemon B, Negrete VF, Davis M, and Korsch BM: Gaps in doctor-patient communication: Doctor-patient interaction analysis. Pediatric Research, *5*:298-311, 1971.

Haynes RB, Taylor DW, and Sackett DL, eds.: *Compliance in Health Care.* Baltimore: Johns Hopkins University Press, 1979.

Haynes RB, Wang E, et al.: A critical review of intervention to improve compliance. Patient Educ. Counsel, *10*:155-66, 1987.

Hulka B: Patient-clinician interactions and compliance. In Haynes RB, Taylor DW, and Sackett DL, eds.: *Compliance in Health Care.* Baltimore: Johns Hopkins University Press, 1979.

Kirscht JP, and Rosenstock IM: Patient problems in following recommendations of health experts. In Stone GC, Cohen F, and Adler NE, eds.: *Health Psychology — A Handbook.* San Francisco. Jossey-Bass, 1979.

Ley P, and Spelman MS: *Communicating with the Patient.* London: Staples Press, 1967.

Maxxullo JC, Lasagna L, and Grinar PF: Variations in interpretation of prescription instructions: The need for improved prescribing habits. JAMA, *224*:929-931, 1974.

McKenney JM, et al.: The effects of clinical pharmacy services on patients with essential hypertension. Circulation. *47*:1104-1111, 1973.

Smith MC: The cost of noncompliance and the capacity of improved compliance to reduce health care expenditures. In *National Pharmaceutical Council: A Symposium.* Reston, VA: National Pharmaceutical Council, 1985.

CHAPTER 9

Communications in Special Situations

OVERVIEW

Applying communication skills to pharmacy practice situations is not always easy. It can be somewhat difficult in situations where patients have special communication needs. These situations require special sensitivities and unique strategies to assure effective communication. This chapter addresses the skills needed to deal with older adults, hearing- and sight-impaired individuals, terminally ill patients, patients with AIDS, patients with mental health problems, adolescents, and individuals taking care of patients ("care givers").

INTRODUCTION

Communication in pharmacy practice is frequently hindered by specific problems surrounding unique types of patients. This chapter discusses specific communication barriers involving a variety of situations. Different strategies are also outlined to assist you in identifying and dealing with these special communication needs.

Before discussing the unique communication problems of these patient groups, one caveat which applies to most situations must be offered: if you sense that a person has a unique problem, you should check your perception of that problem (see Chapter 2). One example is how we typically treat the elderly. Although some elderly patients may appear to be frail, they may not be forgetful or hearing impaired. However, we make certain assumptions based on our perceptions of the elderly as a group of patients. Thus, we start shouting at them and talking slower. The key is to assess how they are responding to our educational efforts. We should watch for nonverbal clues to see if they are leaning towards us or if they have a confused look on their face. Asking open-ended questions can also provide feedback about the patient's ability to communicate. Not checking initial impressions could lead to some potentially embarrassing situations for both patient and pharmacist. Try to avoid stereotyping individuals and make sure to check your perceptions.

OLDER ADULTS

Several factors make it imperative that pharmacists be sensitive to interactions involving older adults. The number of elderly in

our society is increasing and the elderly consume a disproportion-
ate amount of prescription and nonprescription medications compared to other age groups (Elderhealth, 1986). Thus, this growing
segment of the population is in need of our patient counseling
services. Unfortunately, the aging process sometimes affects certain elements of the communication process in some older adults.
These potential communication problems are discussed below.

Learning

In certain individuals the aging process tends to affect the
learning process, but not the ability to learn. Some older adults
learn at a slower rate than younger persons. They have the ability
to learn, but process information at a different rate. Thus, the rate
of speech and the amount of information presented at one time
must meet the individual's ability to comprehend the material. In
addition, short-term memory, recall, and attention span may be
diminished for some elderly patients. The ability to process new
and innovative solutions to problems might also be slower in some
older adults. Thus, attempts to change behaviors should be structured gradually and should build on past experiences. A good approach with some older adults is to set reasonable short-term
goals, approach long-term goals in stages, and break down learning
tasks into smaller components. Another important step is to encourage feedback from patients as to whether they received your
intended message by tactfully asking the patient to repeat instructions and other information and by watching their nonverbal response. When given the opportunity to learn at their own speed,
most of these individuals can learn as well as younger adults.

Vision

Aging may affect the visual process. In some individuals, more
light is needed to stimulate the receptors in the eye. Thus, when
using written information, make sure you have enough light.
Many times visual acuity is not as sharp, and sensitivity to color is
decreased. Written messages for individuals with visual deficiencies should be in large print and on pastel-colored paper rather
than on white paper.

Hearing

Aging may also affect the hearing process. Auditory loss in various degrees of severity is seen in more than one-half of all older adults (Elderhealth, 1986). The hearing loss associated with the aging process is called presbycusis. Unfortunately, this condition may lead to individuals withdrawing socially and psychologically or in extreme cases may lead to them being labeled as senile or forgetful. Many older adults describe their hearing impairment as being able to hear what others are saying, but not being able to understand what is being said. They can hear words, but they cannot put them together clearly.

Other types of hearing loss seen in some older adults are related to the actual hearing process. Response to high-frequency sounds is usually diminished before the response to lower sounds. Thus, using a lower tone of voice may help some older adults. In some older individuals, sensitivity to sound is decreased, and the volume must be increased to stimulate the receptors. It is also important to slow your rate of speech somewhat so that the person can differentiate between the words. As mentioned earlier, it is important not to shout when speaking, because shouting may offend some individuals. Talking in a somewhat higher volume may be necessary, but more likely a slower rate of speech could help most individuals.

Three general types of physical hearing impairment (conductive, sensorineural, and central) can occur singly or in combination with one another (Fox, 1971). Conductive hearing impairment results when something blocks the conduction of sound into the ear's sensory nerve centers. Sensorineural impairment occurs when the problem is situated in the sensory center of the inner ear. Central hearing impairment occurs when the nerve centers that are within the brain are affected. The use of a hearing aid is helpful in conductive hearing problems, but is less effective in sensorineural impairment and is ineffective in central loss. Because the hearing aid only makes the sound louder, it is not too helpful in patients who cannot distinguish sounds easily and may actually make some situations worse. Hearing deficiencies can also be caused by a variety of factors other than the aging process: birth defects, injuries, and chronic exposure to loud noises.

Many individuals with hearing deficiencies, including some older adults, rely on speechreading (watching the lips, facial expressions, and gestures) to enhance their communication ability (Fox, 1971). Speechreading is more than just lipreading. It involves receiving visual cues from facial expressions, body postures, and gestures as well as lip movements. Research has shown that everyone develops some speechreading skill and that the hearing-impaired need to develop that skill much further. Development of this skill is further hindered if patient sight is impaired as well, such as in some older adults. In order for speechreading to be most effective you should position the patient directly in front of you and you should have a light shining on your lips and face when communicating with her.

To improve communication with the hearing-impaired try to position yourself about three to six feet from the patient; never speak directly into the patient's ear, it may distort the message; wait until the patient can see you before speaking; and if necessary, touch her to get her attention. If your message does not appear to be getting through, you should not keep repeating the same statement, but rephrase it in shorter, simpler sentences. Many pharmacists have learned sign language to assist hearing-impaired patients. Finally, you should be aware of environmental barriers, such as loud background noises or dimly lit counseling areas that further make communication difficult for the hearing-impaired.

Value and Perceptual Differences

Another potential communication barrier between you and an older patient may be due to the generation gap. Some older adults may perceive things differently from those in different age groups, because people typically adhere to values learned and accepted in their younger years. Thus, some older adults may have different beliefs and perceptions about health care in general and about drugs and pharmacists specifically. Some behaviors, such as hoarding and sharing medication, may seem inappropriate to you, but such actions may make sense to someone who grew up in the 1930s during the Depression. You should be aware when you may be reacting to their different values and belief systems rather than to patients themselves.

Their image of the pharmacist is also important. They may expect a well-groomed, clean-shaven, professional-looking male practitioner to serve them. If you do not meet these expectations, they may be somewhat reluctant to interact with you initially. Finally, their perception of authority may also influence how they interact with you. Some older adults grew up respecting the authority of physicians and pharmacists and prefer an authoritarian approach to receiving health care. Thus, they may be receptive to being told what to do. On the other hand, other patients may want to be more independent and may feel a need to assert themselves. Thus, they may be somewhat more demanding and may want additional information and more input into the medication decision-making process. Thus, it is important to assess which approach seems to work with each patient.

Psychosocial Factors

Several psychosocial factors may influence your relationship with older adults. First, some older adults may be experiencing a significant amount of loss compared to individuals in other age groups. For example, their friends may be dying at an increased rate; they may have retired from their jobs; or they may have had to slow down or cease certain activities due to the aging process. All of these situations involve loss and subsequent grieving. Thus, their reaction to certain medical situations, such as ignoring your directions or complaining about the price of their medication, may be responses to fear of the disease, of becoming even less active, or of dying. They may deny the situation or become angry at you and other health care providers. They may also turn to self-diagnosis and self-treatment or the use of other people's medications.

SPEECH IMPAIRMENTS AS BARRIERS TO COMMUNICATION

In pharmacy practice, you may need to interact with individuals who have some type of speech impairment or deficiency. Speech deficiencies can be caused by a variety of factors, such as birth defects, injuries, or illnesses (Fox, 1971). A common speech deficiency is dysarthria, or interference with normal control of the speech mechanism. Diseases, such as Parkinson's, multiple sclerosis, and bulbar palsy, as well as strokes and accidents, can cause dysarthria. In dysarthria, speech may be slurred or otherwise difficult to understand due to lack of ability to produce speech sounds correctly, maintain good breath control, or coordinate the movements of the lips, tongue, palate, and larynx. Many of these patients can be helped by using certain medications or by therapy from a trained speech pathologist.

Another common speech problem results from the removal of the larynx secondary to throat cancer or other conditions. These individuals can usually learn to speak again either by learning esophageal speech or by using an electronic device. However, you must be sensitive to these patients, because they sound "different." Many people realize they sound different and that they may make other people feel uncomfortable. Thus, they may shy away from interacting with others.

To overcome these barriers described above, many patients write notes to their pharmacists or use sign language as a means of communicating. Some pharmacists have responded to this need by providing writing pads for patients and by even learning how to sign along with the patient.

Aphasia

A related group of patients with speech difficulties are stroke victims who suffer from aphasia. Aphasia is a complex problem, which may result, to varying degrees, in the reduced ability to understand what others are saying and to express oneself. Some patients may have no speech, while others may have only mild difficulties recalling names or words. Others may have problems putting words in their proper order in a sentence. Speech may be limited to short phrases or single words; or smaller words are left out so that the sentence reads like a telegram. The ability to understand oral directions, to read, to write, and to deal with numbers may also be disturbed. Fortunately, in some patients communication ability can be improved after extensive therapy. However, improvements are often seen in small increments.

Aphasic patients usually have normal hearing acuity; shouting at them will not help. Their problem is one of comprehension; they are not hard of hearing, stubborn, or inattentive. Until you are aware of the extent of language impairment, avoid complex conversations. You should be patient with these individuals when discussing their medications. Many times they will get frustrated with their situation because they know what they want to say but cannot say it. Also it takes longer to communicate with them, because they may hear the word but may not immediately recall the meaning of it. Patience is also needed, because you may want to fill in the word or phrase that the patient is trying to say. It is best to let the patient try. If the patient is unsuccessful after a few attempts, help them by supplying a few words in multiple-choice fashion and let them select the word they desire. Aphasic patients often feel isolated and withdraw from social interactions. Thus, they should be encouraged to interact with other people, and most appreciate being included in a conversation even if only to listen.

Some aphasic patients have difficulty reading. The difficulty is not one of visual acuity but rather of comprehending written language. Some have severe dyslexia and cannot read at all; others can read single words with comprehension but cannot read sentences. Patients with dyslexia may not be able to write notes to you. Dyslexia is not a physical disability but rather the inability to recall or form conventional written symbols.

Many aphasic patients retain certain automatic responses and may appear to be able to communicate very well. They can count up to 10 but may not be able to count four items placed in front of them. They can name the days of the week, but not tell you that Tuesday comes before Thursday. They can function effectively only in repetitive situations. Usually these automatic speech skills are within socially acceptable limits, but sometimes patients utter profanities that may embarrass both the listener and the patient. Patients are not displaying anger or other displeasures when they curse, but rather are using automatic speech and are unable to inhibit these responses. As a pharmacist, you will have difficulty counseling aphasic patients, but as discussed above you should at least make an attempt, because they may benefit from the experience. Although getting feedback from aphasic patients as to whether or not they received the message as you intended may be difficult, that should not prevent you from attempting communication with them. Many times it is best to counsel the person who is caring for the aphasic patient, but do not exclude the patient from this experience.

TERMINALLY ILL PATIENTS

Most individuals, including pharmacists, find it somewhat difficult to interact with terminally ill patients. People typically feel uncomfortable discussing the topic of death and are uncertain about what to say; they do not want to say the "wrong" thing or upset the patient. Yet most terminally ill patients need supportive relationships from family members, friends, and pharmacists.

Pharmacists are becoming increasingly important in the care of terminally ill patients due to the complex nature of cancer therapy and their increased involvement on oncology teams in hospitals and other institutions. By the same token, more community-based pharmacists are getting involved due to the deinstitutionalization of cancer treatment and the evolution of home health care as a popular option for many patients. More importantly, pharmacists may be the only health professional in their community readily accessible to patient and family. Thus, you should be ready, professionally and emotionally, to interact with these patients.

Several communication strategies have been offered by professionals who have worked with the terminally ill. Many of these approaches are too complex to be discussed in detail here but are listed in the recommended readings at the end of this chapter (Beardsley, et al., 1977; Feifel, 1977; Kubler-Ross, 1969). Most strategies require "meeting the patients where they are" in relation to their understanding of their condition and their stage of adjustment. For example, a patient may be denying the existence of her illness, or she may be angry or depressed about her situation. You would approach these two situations differently. The key is to ask open-ended questions, such as "How are you doing today?" or "How are things going?" to determine the patient's willingness to discuss the situation with you. You should not assume that the patient does not want to talk about it. Even if patients do not respond initially, they at least realize you are willing to talk and may open up at a later time.

Before interacting with terminally ill patients, you must be aware of your own feelings about death and interacting with terminally ill patients. Do you typically avoid conversations with these patients? Do they remind you of a friend's or a family member's struggle with a terminal illness? Being aware of your feelings will help you assist these patients. You should realize which cases should be referred to others for assistance and which ones you can handle yourself. Many pharmacists have found that just being honest about their feelings improves their interaction with terminally ill patients. Just by saying "I don't know what to say right now, but how are you doing?" or "I feel so helpless. Is there anything I can do for you?" seems to communicate your concern for the patient and gives her a chance to share her concerns as well. As in any type of patient interaction, the degree of involvement depends on your relationship with the patient. You will be more open with some patients than with others. It is also important to implicitly or explicitly set limits on what you can do for the patient. You must communicate your concern without raising patient expectations that you can assist in all areas of her life.

Many terminally ill patients realize they make other people feel uncomfortable, and they tend to avoid interactions. However, if you can express your uneasiness or your frustration about not knowing how to help them at the same time that you express your concern for them, patients will typically feel more at ease and more willing to express their own feelings.

You may also come in contact with family members who have special needs. Research has shown that family members go through the same type of stages as dying patients and thus need support and often drug therapy (Kubler-Ross, 1969). As with the terminally ill patients, you may be called upon to be a good listener to lend support to the family members.

In summary, as pharmacists, communication with terminally ill patients and their families is extremely important. You should not avoid talking with them unless you sense that they do not want to talk about their illness. Not interacting with them only contributes further to their isolation and may reaffirm the idea that talking about death is uncomfortable.

PATIENTS WITH AIDS

Due to the increased prevalence of AIDS and the unique characteristics of this disease, pharmacists must be prepared to assist patients with AIDS. Not only are these individuals dealing with a potentially life-threatening disease, they are also dealing with the social stigma which many times accompanies the disease. The key is not to treat them as being "different" from your other patients. But typically, they do have a unique set of needs which must be recognized and addressed. Many of the issues discussed above in the terminally ill section apply to AIDS patients because obviously AIDS is a type of terminal disease. Many have the same needs as other terminally ill patients. Thus, you should use some of the strategies outlined above, such as using open-ended questions to determine patient receptivity to interaction.

However, patients with AIDS have special needs which should be considered. For example, many patients are without an adequate support system because relationships with family and friends are somewhat strained due to the social stigma. You may be asked to be part of the patient's support system or may be called upon to refer the patient to an appropriate source of support. You may need to supply additional triage or problem-solving support because others are not providing it. Many patients have trouble dealing with their own -identity as the disease progresses. In many cases, dealing with AIDS has a physical component (i.e., weight loss, lack of energy), but also psychological and sociological aspects (i.e., becoming more dependent on others, fear of dying, fear of pain). They are wrestling with a lot of issues and may need some assistance sorting things out.

Patients must also deal with misinformation and inaccurate perceptions about AIDS. Many people around them do not understand the various aspects of the disease or its treatment. Hopefully, pharmacists are not included in this misinformed group. We must keep up with the latest literature, because we know that most AIDS patients certainly monitor what is being researched.

In working with patients with AIDS, pharmacists must first evaluate their attitudes towards this disease and the patients who have it. They may be reacting to their perception of these patients as a group rather than to patients as individuals in need of help. Pharmacists need to recognize the potential biases which may prevent them from interacting with patients. At the same time, pharmacists must determine what their role should be in assisting patients. Many pharmacists feel comfortable becoming close members of patient support networks and taking an active role in assuring that patient needs are met. The key is to identify what the patient needs and what services you can provide to best meet them.

PATIENTS WITH MENTAL HEALTH PROBLEMS

Many pharmacists admit that they have difficulty communicating with another unique group of patients: those with mental health disorders. By the same token, many mental health patients may be reluctant to interact with other individuals.

Some pharmacists feel that they do not know what to say to these patients. They are afraid of saying the wrong thing or saying something that might cause an emotional outburst by the patient in the pharmacy. Some pharmacists are also unsure of how much information they should provide to such patients about their condition and treatment. Many times it is unclear what patients already understand about their condition and what their physicians have told them. Once again, open-ended questions are good tools to use to determine the level of patient understanding before you counsel them about the medication. Examples include, "What has the doctor told you about this medication?" or "This drug can be used for many things. What has your physician said?" Asking open-ended questions also helps you determine patient cognitive functioning, that is, are they able to comprehend what you are saying and can they articulate their concerns to you? If they cannot, you may have to communicate through a care giver or someone else. Some pharmacists may also be reluctant to distribute written information to patients receiving psychotropic medications for fear that patients may misinterpret the information. Another related concern is that many psychotropic medications, such as imipramine for bed wetting and diazepam for muscle spasms, are used for nonmental health disorders. Thus, the written material may not be relevant to the patient's condition and may only cause alarm. It is important that all material be carefully screened prior to distribution and that you make an attempt to reinforce the information verbally to assure a better understanding by the patient.

Pharmacists interacting with patients with mental disorders must address a more fundamental ethical issue: should patients with mental disorders be allowed the same level of information regarding their drug treatment and the same type of informed consent as patients with nonpsychiatric disorders? Does the uniqueness of having a mental illness versus a physical illness preclude them from knowing more about the effects (both positive and negative) of their drugs? Do we withhold certain information that would be given to a nonpsychiatric patient? Obviously, each situation must be evaluated individually and many times in consultation with the patient's physician. However, the point is raised here because how you deal with these questions will affect how you communicate with mental health patients. Many pharmacists have developed tactful ways of addressing patient concerns, while at the same time not suggesting things that may interfere with treatment. In some situations, trusting relationships may develop between patient, practitioner, and pharmacist. In these cases, the pharmacists can be completely open with patients and even serve as part of their case management team.

Unfortunately, certain stereotypes about mental illness and patients with these disorders tend to inhibit communication. Society in general, as well as many pharmacists, has certain stigmas and misconceptions about mental illness. We tend to categorize people based on images from the media or from our past perceptions about how "crazy" people act. Our reluctance is also reinforced by the fact that some patients indeed act "different." They may have awkward body and facial movements (possibly due to their medications). Some are chronic cigarette smokers and have poor hygienic habits. They may say what we think are bizarre statements. They may not make good eye contact, which may make us even more uncomfortable.

Patients may be reluctant to interact with pharmacists for a variety of reasons. First, they may have a poor self-concept and may be insecure about interacting with others. They may also realize that they have a condition that makes other people uncomfortable.

Thus, this societal stigma about mental illness makes them avoid social interactions. In some cases, patients may be paranoid about dealing with other people, especially health care professionals. Thus, your attempts to communicate with these patients may find initial patient resistance. Patients typically need multiple contacts to establish trusting relationships. However, you should realize that this may never happen and that your interactions may always be "different," compared to your relationships with other patients. But, these differences should be handled the same way that you deal with other unique individuals discussed in previous section. Differences should not stop you from trying to interact with these special patients. However, these potential communication problems may require you to be innovative in developing strategies to overcome them.

ADOLESCENTS

Adolescents are a unique group of individuals in a variety of ways. They are dealing with so many issues in their lives (physical changes, independence/dependence, -identity). Because they also may be dealing with new health issues (acne, menstrual problems, sexual activity), it is important to recognize how pharmacists can assist them with their health needs. Unfortunately, many pharmacists confess that it is difficult to interact with this age group. In order to improve communication with adolescents, Dolinsky and Werner (1987) offer the following considerations:

1. Adolescents may become self-preoccupied, believing that they are the center of other people's attention.

2. Peer groups play an important role in their decision-making process.

3. They may resent being told what to do (need to become more independent) and will not ask for help (will not admit that they do not understand something). However, stressful events, such as an illness, may cause them to revert back to more dependent behavior.

4. Adolescents do not react to symptoms of pain or illness. They may ignore important signs of disease.

5. Many have the perception that "nobody understands me," which may include pharmacists as well.

Strategies to improve communications include: 1) using empathy (give the perception that you are really trying to listen, understand and help), 2) communicating that you accept them as they are, 3) using open-ended questions to draw their real feelings out, and 4) using innovative written material to convey health messages in relevant terms and expressions. In recent years, clever, accurate material has been developed for drug abuse, cigarette smoking, sexually transmitted diseases, and birth control.

In summary, pharmacists can improve communication with adolescents by applying the general communication skills discussed in previous chapters (empathy, open-ended questioning, and listening) to this set of individuals. Pharmacists need to be sincere about their interactions; they do not have to act like adolescents or use their language in order to interact with them. They must convey a feeling of understanding and acceptance while providing information.

CARE GIVERS

Several special communication problems arise when pharmacists need to interact with patient care givers rather than patients themselves. Care givers can be individuals who take care of older adults with chronic conditions or parents who take care of children during acute illnesses. They can be family members, friends, or hired assistants. In general, the number of these care givers will probably increase in the future, because there has been an increased effort to shift patient care from hospitals to home care. Dealing with care givers takes a set of specific strategies, because you cannot communicate directly with the patient and thus cannot determine if the patient received your intended message. It is also difficult to assess patient compliance and to offer support and encouragement to the patient regarding drug treatment.

When dealing with care givers, certain areas should be addressed. First, care givers need to understand the patient's condition and treatment, and how to communicate specific instructions to the patient. The care giver must also understand how to monitor the patient's therapeutic response to a specific medication, how to monitor for adverse drug events, and how to report any suspicious events. They should be instructed on the importance of good nutrition and fluid intake for certain types of patients. They must be reminded about the refill status of the medication and when the physician needs to be contacted. They should be encouraged to contact you if they have any questions or if the patient has specific questions.

Written information about the medication is essential, because the message should be delivered to the patient. A follow-up phone call to the patient may also be necessary to make sure that the message was received and to reinforce key points regarding drug therapy. Many pharmacists use medication reminder systems (i.e., drug calendars, weekly medication containers) to help the care giver keep track of the patient's medication.

In addition, you should develop a special sensitivity to care givers and should not merely view them as someone picking up the medication for the patient. Many times, the care givers have special needs themselves. They may be under a lot of stress trying to care for the patient at home. They may have careers and other activities outside the home and may be financially strained as well. Serious depression has been found in almost one-fourth of the individuals caring for the home-bound elderly. In some situations, the care givers may be patients themselves with their own medical problems. It is interesting to note that one of the fastest-growing segments of our population is the group of people over 65 with parents in their 80s and 90s (Elderhealth, 1986). Thus, two generations of patients with health problems may be living in the same home. You should also respond empathically to the care giver and try to understand some of their personal problems. As mentioned earlier, pharmacists are often the most accessible health care professional in the community and may be the only consistent contact a care giver has with the health care network. You should be aware of the care giver's nonverbal messages and must not be afraid to ask, "What is on your mind?"

You should also be aware of the different support groups in the community that could assist the care givers, such as local hospice organizations for terminally ill patients at home.

SUMMARY

Pharmacists will always be challenged by situations needing special attention. Although the groups discussed in this chapter do not represent the entire universe of patients with special communication needs, they do reflect the majority of groups that deserve special consideration in pharmacy practice. Pharmacists need to first recognize patients with special communication needs and then develop effective strategies to overcome these specific barriers to the communication process.

REFERENCES

Beardsley RS, Johnson CA, Benson SB: Pharmacists' interaction with the terminally ill patient, J. Am Pharm Assoc, *NS17*:750-752, 1977.

Dolinsky D, Werner K: How to counsel the adolescent patient. Drug Topics, May 4, 1987:69-75.

Elderhealth: Consumer drug education program. MD Pharm., *62*:4, 1986.

Feifel H: *New Meanings of Death.* New York: McGraw-Hill, 1977.

Fox MJ: Talking with patients who can't answer. Am. J. Nursing, *71*:1146-1148, 1971.

Kubler-Ross E: *On Death and Dying.* New York: Macmillan, 1969.

RECOMMENDED READINGS

Bird B: *Talking with Patients.* 2nd ed. Philadelphia: JB Lippincott, 1973.

Communicating with the Elderly: Pharmacy Practice for the Geriatric Patient. Alexandria, VA: American Association of Colleges of Pharmacy, 1985.

Communication Problems and Behaviors of Older Americans. Rockville, MD: American Speech-Language-Hearing Association, 1979.

CHAPTER *10*

Ethical Patient Care

OVERVIEW

Pharmacists, as health professionals, have ethical obligations to patients and to society. In order to know how to resolve moral dilemmas and make ethical decisions, pharmacists must understand general ethical principles and their applications in pharmaceutical care situations. This chapter outlines key principles relevant to pharmacist-patient relationships, and presents a decision-making process to assist pharmacists in resolving ethical conflicts.

ETHICAL PATIENT CARE

Case #1

A patient who is being started on a new medication asks you questions about the purpose of the medication and possible side effects. When you ask him what his physician told him about the medication, it is obvious to you that he is unclear as to its purpose or possible problems.

The drug does have a number of side effects, some of which can be serious. The patient reports that when he asked his physician about side effects, the physician replied, "I have many patients on this drug and they're doing fine." You are concerned that the patient may refuse to take the drug if told about possible side effects.

Case #2

In response to OBRA '90 legislation, the management of the pharmacy you work for has trained the clerks in the organization to say to patients in a neutral tone of voice "Do you wish to receive counseling from the pharmacist?" You argue that this approach is inadequate and you want to talk with patients personally. You insist that this is the only way you can verify that they understand how to use their medications and are aware of potential problems. The manager says that counseling is not required under OBRA when the patient declines the offer to discuss. Furthermore, he says, the store is too busy to go beyond the minimum legally required and is financially having trouble surviving the intense competition in the area as it is. He goes on to state that he encourages pharmacists to counsel patients in depth if the pharmacist has time and there are no other patients waiting for their prescriptions.

Case #3

James Bently, a 16-year-old patient of your pharmacy, was recently diagnosed with epilepsy and prescribed phenytoin. In conversations with him, you have discovered that he considers epilepsy embarrassing and has indicated that he doesn't believe his physician is correct in the diagnosis. Your refill records indicate a pattern of noncompliance, which the patient has confirmed by expressing his belief that he does not really need the drug. You have extensively educated him about phenytoin and the importance of consistent use in controlling seizures, but he continues to be noncompliant. He also continues to drive his car and was recently charged in a non-injury automobile accident. His father, who picked up a recent prescription for James, has never indicated awareness of his son's denial of epilepsy or noncompliance with treatment. Should you disclose to the father the fact that James is noncompliant? How about the police? his physician?

Each of these patient cases presents the pharmacist with a decision that has, at its core, ethical dimensions. The pharmacist's ability to choose a proper course of action in these situations depends on his understanding of the principles underlying the ethical treatment of patients by health professionals. A discussion of these principles and the situations in which they apply in pharmacy practice will be presented in this chapter. The development of an individual's ability to make moral judgments will also be described. Finally, a decision-making process which pharmacists can use to assess ethical situations as they arise and to reach ethical decisions will be outlined.

Principles that have been recognized as underlying ethics in medical decision making include: beneficence, autonomy and honesty (Beauchamp & Childers, 1989; Van de Veer & Regan, 1987; Veatch, 1981; Veatch, 1989a). Other values which derive from these principles and are particularly important in health care are informed consent, confidentiality, and fidelity. While this is by no means a complete list, these principles seem to be most relevant to the communication responsibilities of pharmacists.

ETHICAL PRINCIPLES

Beneficence

Beneficence is the principle that health professionals should act in the best interest of the patient. The principle of beneficence is found in the Hippocratic Oath, which states that the physician will apply measures "for the benefit of the sick according to my ability and judgment." The APhA code of ethics (Buerki, 1985) has a section based on the beneficence principle which states "A pharmacist should hold the health and safety of the patient to be of first consideration and should render to each patient the full measure of professional ability as an essential health practitioner."

Unfortunately, the history of medicine has used the beneficence principle as justification for a "paternalistic" relationship with patients. Under a paternalistic ethic, physicians made decisions by themselves (without necessarily informing patients and without patient consent) as to what was in the patient's best interest.

More recent work in medical ethics has highlighted the dangers of beneficence — dangers that threaten the core of our political philosophy, which emphasizes individual rights and personal liberties. These rights, by extension, include the right to decide for oneself whether treatment is or is not in one's own best interest.

Autonomy

The principle of autonomy establishes a patient's right to self-determination — to choose what will be done to his person. This right is considered paramount even if a health professional may judge a patient's decision as being damaging to his health. The value of self-determination is seen as independent of the outcome of one's autonomous choice.

Honesty

The honesty principle states that patients have the right to the truth about their medical condition, the course of their disease, treatments recommended, and alternative treatments available. The APhA code of ethics states that a pharmacist "should strive to provide information to patients regarding professional services truthfully, accurately and fully."

Informed Consent

Both honesty and autonomy serve as foundations to the patient's right to give informed consent to treatment. The informed consent principle states that patients have the right to full disclosure of all relevant aspects of care and must give explicit consent to treatment before treatment is initiated. Typically, informed consent is presented as consisting of five components: disclosure, comprehension, voluntariness, competence, and consent (Brock, 1987; Beauchamp, 1989).

If all relevant information is provided; if the patient understands the information; if consent is freely given if the patient is capable of understanding the salient information and, with that understanding, coming to a decision; and if the patient gives consent to a particular treatment, then informed consent has occurred and treatment can be implemented.

Unfortunately, in practice the right of the patient to provide informed consent has resulted in actions by health professionals which focus more on "disclosure" than on patient understanding. The term "informed consent" has come to be equated with the "consent forms" patients are required to sign before initiation of some types of medical treatment (e.g., surgery). However, a shift in focus in the informed consent literature is now emphasizing the quality of a patient's understanding as a more essential component than disclosure per se. Beauchamp (1989) summarizes this position and states that "the central problems about informed consent are issues of communication rather than the abstract and disembodied issues about proper legal standards of disclosure." He goes on to state that "the key to effective communication is to invite participation by patients or subjects in an exchange of information and disclosure. Asking questions, eliciting the concerns and interests of the patient or subject, and establishing a climate that encourages the patient or subject to ask questions may be more important than the full corpus of disclosed information."

It is not sufficient, given the above definition of informed consent, for the health professional to be "available" to consult or respond to questions. A meaningful dialogue or consent process is unlikely to be initiated by patients themselves for a variety of reasons. This is true, in part, due to patient reticence to question providers. In addition, patients often cannot *know* when there is important information about treatment that they have not yet acquired. The burden is on the health care professional to make *sure* patients understand all they need to know to both make a reasoned decision about therapy and to implement therapeutic plans appropriately.

What is the role of the pharmacist in informed consent? Pharmacists seem to function under the assumption that, when a patient brings in a prescription, a) the physician has provided all relevant information, b) the patient has understood the information, and c) the patient has consented to treatment. In fact, research strongly suggests than none of these assumptions may be true. Often, patients have been found to misunderstand or lack information on crucial aspects of drug treatment (Ley, 1983; Semla, et al., 1991). In addition, physicians frequently do not explicitly discuss key aspects of drug therapy (Svarstad, 1976) and often fail to obtain meaningful consent from patients (Lidz, et al., 1983; Wu & Perlman, 1988). If it is a pharmacist's responsibility to verify the patient's understanding of a medication, including its purpose, appropriate use, possible side effects, and so on, then in the course of such an assessment it may become obvious that informed consent has really *not* occurred. The patient may not fully understand important aspects of treatment, may have unanswered questions, may not be aware of significant side effects — all of which would indicate that informed consent to treatment is not present. In addition, the patient may indicate reluctance to begin taking the medication but feel that he has no choice except to do as the physician says. The question of what constitutes "coercion," given a relationship where power is largely vested in health professionals upon whom patients feel dependent, is critical in determining if consent to treatment has been freely given. When a patient expresses reservations about initiating drug treatment, it may be necessary for the pharmacist to consult not only with the patient but also with the prescribing physician to inform him of the lack of freely given consent to treatment.

It is, perhaps, ironic that surgery has been the prototype for issues of informed consent, whereas drug therapy has been largely ignored. Drug treatment is a more pervasive form of treatment than is surgery; the patient has much more control over management of therapy (although not, perhaps, greater participation in original decisions to treat); and estimates of the costs to society of medication-related illness are staggering (Hepler & Strand, 1990). The assumption in society appears to be that the risks associated with drug therapy are minimal. With increased attention to the problems created by inappropriate therapy (including inappropriate combinations of drugs) and misuse of medications, these assumptions of minimal risk will likely change, and pharmacists will undoubtedly be expected to assume their share of responsibility as health care professionals in assuring that informed consent has occurred before treatment is initiated.

Confidentiality

This principle serves to assure patients that information about their medical conditions and treatments will not be given to third parties without their permission. Brody (1989) makes the case that confidentiality is "central to preserving the human dignity of patients." He explains that a large part of our personal sense of control over our lives is wrapped up in our ability to choose to whom we wish to reveal our most personal selves and what information we wish to confide. Self-disclosure is the essence of intimacy in relationships and we desire control over this most personal act.

The relationship between patient and health provider circumvents the normal progression of intimate relationships. Patients are expected to divulge the most personal details of their existence to virtual strangers. To maintain the reciprocal trust that is essential in these relationships, professionals must be able to trust the truthfulness of patient reports and patients must be able to trust that this information will not be shared with others not involved in their medical care.

Fidelity

Fidelity is the right of patients to have health professionals provide services that promote the patient's interest rather than those that serve a competing or conflicting interest. A pharmacist who encourages the use of vitamins the patient does not need may be promoting his financial well-being at the expense of the patient. A pharmacist who refuses to confront a physician about inappropriate prescribing because he wants to ensure that the physician will continue to direct patients to his pharmacy is displaying a misplaced sense of professional responsibility. The pharmacist who is more attentive to the desires of the party signing his paycheck than to the health care needs of his patients is in a conflict of interest situation. Ethically, the responsibility of a health professional is, first and foremost, to the welfare of the patient.

THE PATIENT-PROVIDER RELATIONSHIP

The focus on the rights of the patient and obligations of the provider can make the relationship between them seem mechanistic and legalistic. However, the true ability to effectively meet these ethical responsibilities is dependent upon a trusting, caring relationship between patient and provider. Fried (1974) identifies four rights that patients have in relationships with health care professionals. In addition to lucidity (the right to full, understandable disclosure), autonomy, and fidelity, he identifies a fourth right which he calls "humanity." Humanity means that the patient has the right to be treated with compassion. Each patient is a unique individual and, in an illness situation, is particularly vulnerable. Patients need humane, sensitive care from providers — care that will assist them in making the best decisions they are able to make in their lives. This is the essence of the "helping" role of the health care professional. Brody (1992) makes the case that the vulnerability of the patient and the status accorded physicians and other health professionals sets up a power difference fraught with danger for the patient. He states that "if one shares the power precisely with the person in greatest danger of being victimized, the potential for self-correction of error seems greatest." Once again, the need for mutual participation and an active patient role in health care decision making becomes essential. Empowering patients to be active participants in treatment decisions, with decisions being made in the context of a respectful, trusting relationship, is a large part of our professional responsibility to patients.

DEVELOPMENT OF MORAL REASONING

Ethical and clinical decision making as a health professional and moral choice outside the professional role are highly interrelated. Ethical and moral decisions, whether professional or personal, occur in the context of our relationships with others. Research has established that a correlation exists between moral reasoning and clinical decision-making by health professionals (Sheehan, et al., 1980). In addition, Self and colleagues (1992, 1989) have found that formal instruction in medical ethics results in higher levels of moral reasoning for general situations as well (). Children have been found to predictably move through stages of moral reasoning which are characterized by changes in the process of making moral decisions. These stages are consonant with the successive stages of cognitive development identified by Piaget (1965; Piaget & Inhelder, 1969) — stages characterized by increasing differentiation of self and others and the development of logical/hypothetical thinking. Kohlberg (1976, 1984, 1986) identified six stages of moral reasoning that he postulates individuals go through in an invariant developmental sequence — stages characterized by increasing moral adequacy of the means of making judgments and resolving moral dilemmas. The six stages of moral reasoning he described are grouped into three levels as follows:

PRECONVENTIONAL LEVEL

Stage 1   Moral Realism

An individual is seen to act in order to avoid breaking rules. The moral significance of an action is seen as inherent in the act itself; punishment is important because it identifies what is "bad," with all people judging any act in the same way.

Stage 2   Individualistic, Instrumental Morality

Individuals are thought to follow rules when there is something in it for them. The rightness of an act becomes defined in terms of what is an equal exchange or what is agreed to in a "deal." Awareness is beginning to emerge that the interests of individuals can differ and therefore conflict.

Conventional Level

Stage 3   Interpersonally Normative Morality

Individuals are thought to act in order to try to live up to what is expected by people close to them. "Being good" is important and includes showing concern for others and maintaining interpersonal relationships.

Stage 4   Social System Morality

Individuals are thought to act in order to fulfill duties to which they have agreed (i.e., meet obligations). What is "right" is understood in terms of what is in the best interest of the society, group, or institution to which one belongs. Moral judgments are made in reference to institutions or systems, whether legal/societal systems or religious institutions.

Postconventional or Principled Level

Stage 5   Human Rights and Social Contract Morality

Society is seen as creating a social system to protect the rights of all members. Laws are based on a "greatest good for the greatest number" perspective. Some rights, however such as "life" and "liberty" are seen as necessary to uphold, regardless of majority opinion.

Stage 6   Universal Ethical Principles

Persons are thought to act in accordance with self-chosen ethical principles which are the "universal" principles of justice, the equality of human rights, and respect for the dignity of human beings as individual persons. People are seen as having value in themselves rather than as agents of societal values.

Kohlberg's theory is not without critics (see Modgil & Modgil, 1986, for a review and critique). Gilligan and her colleagues (1977, 1982, 1988) charge that Kohlberg's theory and method of assessing development in moral reasoning was based on research with boys and men. The more advanced stages in Kohlberg's theory hold "justice" as the key principle for making ethical decisions. Gilligan contends that girls, while being able to use a justice orientation in moral reasoning, tend to preferentially use reasoning based on what she calls a "caring" principle. This orientation stresses an individual's responsibilities in relationships with others and strives for solutions responsive to the needs of all the individuals involved. However, research on Kohlberg's theory of moral reasoning (see Rest, 1986, for a review) has generally failed to find differences based on gender. These findings negate Gilligan's assertion that the Kohlberg theory is biased against women but do not invalidate her assertion that an alternative moral code focusing on interpersonal responsibilities can be seen as a fully principled code. Rest, whose theoretical work has built on Kohlberg's research, has examined personal and environmental variables related to development of moral judgment and moral behavior (Rest, 1986). In summarizing the results of hundreds of studies he has reviewed, he concludes that "the people who develop in moral judgment are those who love to learn, who seek new challenges, who enjoy intellectually stimulating environments, who are reflective … who take responsibility for themselves and their environs … who operate in social milieus that support their work, endeavor to interest them, and reward their accomplishment … [who] are more fulfilled in their career aspirations … are more involved in their communities, and take more interest in the larger societal issues." The extent to which pharmacy colleges, work settings and other professional institutions foster environments that reward intellectual striving and professional challenge may be the extent to which these institutions facilitate the moral and ethical growth of pharmacists. Conversely, if environments stifle or fail to reward such aspirations, they inhibit continued growth of pharmacists as ethical health professionals.

RESOLVING ETHICAL DILEMMAS

The Decision-Making Process

The steps involved in reaching an ethical decision are essentially identical for resolving either professional/ethical or general moral dilemmas. These steps are summarized below.

1. Recognize and state the ethical dilemma(s) involved in a situation or case.

2. Collect all of the relevant facts. The facts include both medical as well as social/psychological aspects of the case that may be relevant. These facts may clarify whether the problem really does involve ethical issues or not.

3. If the problem involves ethical issues, generate all possible alternatives to resolving the ethical dilemma.

4. Evaluate alternatives in terms of principles that apply as well as possible consequences of the different choices. One exercise that is useful is to provide principle-based justification for all alternatives, arguing on either side of an ethical dilemma.

5. Choose the best alternative (or combine alternatives) and justify your choice in terms of the prioritization of ethical principles involved. Often one principle must be suspended in favor of a more compelling principle in resolving a dilemma.

6. Recommend a specific course of action.

ANALYZING PATIENT CASES

The chapter began with a description of three patient cases that presented ethical dilemmas to pharmacists. These cases will now be analyzed according to the competing ethical principles that are involved.

Case #1

When the patient does not understand the purpose of drug treatment or the possible side effects that may occur, it is obvious that he has not, in fact, given informed consent to treatment. The argument in favor of having the pharmacist provide him with information about the medication, including its purpose and side effects, involves respect for the patient's autonomy and his right to determine what will be done to his body. The pharmacist may have to call the physician to gather further information pertinent to this patient's treatment and may consult with the physician on how to assure that informed consent takes place. Nevertheless, the decision would be that the patient has the right to this information and must be informed before he begins taking the medication.

Arguments against providing information may revolve around fears that the patient may not take medications he needs to treat his medical condition if he is aware of the side effects. The principle invoked in such a case is beneficence — doing something which the pharmacist decides is in the patient's best interest.

Other arguments against informing the patient may focus on the physician — on beliefs that it is the physician's responsibility to inform patients, or the physician's right to choose not to provide the patient with certain information about his treatment. Other arguments may focus on the pharmacist's fears about antagonizing physicians by acting contrary to their wishes and jeopardizing physician referrals to the pharmacy.

These latter concerns clearly have the pharmacist in a conflict-of-interest situation where self-interest or allegiances to others (e.g., physicians) are allowed to override the interests of the patient. The right of the patient to fidelity in relationship with the pharmacist is threatened by such a position.

While the principles of beneficence and autonomy may be in conflict in this case, the right of self-determination by the patient is so fundamental as to be paramount. In this case, the patient has the right to information about his medication regardless of whether that information would affect his decision to initiate treatment.

Case #2

The pharmacist whose manager wishes him to curtail patient counseling activities is clearly in a conflict-of-interest situation. The pharmacist's self-interest (pleasing his boss, keeping his job) is pitted against the patient's need for information about prescribed medications.

One of the defining characteristics of health professionals is that they hold the needs of patients above all else. Furthermore, the way in which pharmacists choose to allocate their time essentially involves ethical decision making. Whenever the amount of consultation provided a patient is based on considerations *other* than patient need (e.g., I was too busy, there were too many other patients waiting), the decision contravenes ethical principles supposedly upheld by health professionals.

Case #3

This case involves a decision on whether or not to reveal confidential information (that the patient is not compliant with his anti-seizure medication regimen). The injunction against release of information without patient consent is strongly held and based in part on the patient's right of self-determination. It is up to the patient to decide what information about his medical treatment is provided to people not involved in his care. The argument for breaking confidentiality probably rests on the principle of beneficence (acting in the best interests of the patient by preventing him from injuring himself in an automobile accident). In fact, in this case, the pharmacist may justify breaking confidentiality by invoking a duty to protect innocent people (e.g., those potentially injured in an automobile accident caused by the patient).

A decision to break confidentiality would obviously be involved where the parents or law enforcement officials are to be informed, but what of informing the prescribing physician? Informing the physician would not constitute a breach of confidentiality because he initiated treatment and medical information can legitimately be shared with other health professionals involved in the patient's care.

Given this analysis, what would your decision be about breaking the confidentiality of James' prescription records by informing his parents or law enforcement officials?

Case #4

To give you more practice in analyzing ethical situations, here is an additional case to analyze:

You are working as a relief pharmacist in a community pharmacy. You notice that the pharmacy has filled prescriptions called in by a physician for the 17-year-old daughter of a very close family friend of yours. One is a refill prescription for oral contraceptives and one is for treatment of a sexually transmitted disease (STD). The girl has been running with a fast crowd and has a boyfriend of whom her parents disapprove and whom they have forbidden her to see. The boyfriend also has a prescription, called in by the same physician, for treatment of an STD. You are very concerned about the girl and wonder whether her use of oral contraceptives may lead her to forego the use of condoms, which could offer protection from STDs. When she comes in to pick up the prescriptions, she becomes upset at seeing you and hurries out, refusing to talk to you. You know that, if you were in her parents' shoes, you would want to know about the prescriptions. You are convinced that the girl is in trouble and needs the help of her family. You are trying to decide whether or not to inform her parents of the prescriptions.

Consider the following questions.

1. What is the ethical dilemma?

2. What additional facts may be needed to help you reach a decision in this case?

3. What alternatives might you consider in resolving the dilemma?

4. What ethical principles are involved in the decision?

5. What alternative would you choose and why?

6. How would you proceed in carrying out your decision?

SUMMARY

Pharmacists must understand the principles that serve as foundations for ethical decisions in health care. The obligation to respect patient autonomy, to protect confidentiality of patient information, to serve the patient's welfare, and to treat patients with respect and compassion are fundamental duties for any health professional. Use of a systematic decision-making process when ethical dilemmas arise and principles seem to compete can assist pharmacists in reaching decisions that are morally valid.

REFERENCES

Beauchamp T: Informed consent. In Veatch RM, ed.: *Medical Ethics.* Boston: Jones and Bartlett, 1989.

Beauchamp TL, and Childers JF: *Principles of Biomedical Ethics.* New York: Oxford University Press, 1989.

Brock DW: Informed consent. In Van de Veer D, and Regan T, eds.: *Health Care Ethics.* Philadelphia: Temple University Press, 1987.

Brody H: *The Healer's Power.* New Haven, CT: Yale University Press, 1992.

Brody H: The physician/patient relationship. In Veatch RM, ed.: *Medical Ethics.* Boston: Jones and Bartlett, 1989.

Buerki RA: *The Challenge of Ethics in Pharmacy Practice.* Madison, WI: American Institute of the History of Pharmacy, 1985.

Fried C: *Medical Experimentation: Personal Integrity and Social Policy.* New York: American Elsevier, 1974.

Gilligan C, Ward JV, and Taylor JM: *Mapping the Moral Domain: A Contribution of Women's Thinking to Psychological Theory and Education.* Cambridge, MA: Harvard University Press, 1988.

Gilligan C: *In a Different Voice: Psychological Theory and Women's Development.* Cambridge, MA: Harvard University Press, 1982.

Gilligan C: In a different voice: Women's conception of the self and of morality. Harvard Educational Review, *47,* 481-517, 1977.

Hepler CD, and Strand LM: Opportunities and responsibilities in pharmaceutical care. American Journal of Hospital Pharmacy, *47,* 533-543, 1990.

Kohlberg L: A current statement on some theoretical issues. In Modgil S, and Modgil C, eds.: *Lawrence Kohlberg: Consensus and Controversy.* Philadelphia: The Falmer Press, 1986.

Kohlberg L: *Essays on Moral Development. Vol. 2: The Psychology of Moral Development.* San Francisco: Harper and Row, 1984.

Kohlberg L: Moral stages and moralization: The cognitive developmental approach. In Lickona T, ed.: *Moral Development and Behavior: The-*

ory, Research and Social Issues. New York: Holt, Rinehart and Winston, 1976.

Ley P: Patients' understanding and recall in clinical communication failure. In Pendleton D, and Hasler J, eds.: *Doctor-Patient Communication.* London: Academic Press, 1983.

Lidz CW, Meisel A, Osterweis M, Holden JL, Marx JH, and Munetz MR: Barriers to informed consent. Annals of Internal Medicine, *99*:539-543, 1983.

Modgil S, and Modgil C: *Lawrence Kohlberg: Consensus and Controversy.* Philadelphia: The Falmer Press, 1986.

Piaget J, and Inhelder B: *The Psychology of the Child.* New York; Basic Books, Inc., 1969.

Piaget J: *The Moral Judgment of the Child.* New York: The Free Press, 1965.

Rest JR: *Moral Development: Advances in Research and Theory.* New York: Praeger, 1986.

Self DJ, Baldwin CJ, and Wolinsky FD: Evaluation of teaching medical ethics by an assessment of moral reasoning. Medical Education, *26*:178-184, 1992.

Self DJ, Wolinsky FD, and Baldwin DC: The effect of teaching medical ethics on medical students' moral reasoning. Academic Medicine, *64*:755-759, 1989.

Semla TP, Lemke JH, Helling DK, Wallace RB, and Chrischilles EA: Perceived purpose of prescription drugs: The Iowa 65+ rural health study. DICP: Annals of Pharmacotherapy, *25*:410-413, 1991.

Sheehan TJ, Husted SDR, Candee D, Cook CD, and Bargen M: Moral judgment as a predictor of clinical performance. Evaluation and the Health Professions, *3*:393-404, 1980.

Svarstad B: Physician-patient communication and patient conformity with medical advice. In Mechanic D, ed.: *The Growth of Bureaucratic Medicine.* New York: John Wiley and Sons, 1976.

Van de Veer D, and Regan T, eds.: *Health Care Ethics.* Philadelphia: Temple University Press, 1987.

Veatch RM, ed.: *Medical Ethics.* Boston: Jones and Bartlett, 1989a.

Veatch RM: *A Theory of Medical Ethics.* New York: Basic Books, Inc., 1981.

Veatch RM: Informed consent: The emerging principles In Wertheimer AI, and Smith MC, eds.,: *Pharmacy Practice: Social and Behavioral Aspects*, 3rd ed., p. 338. Baltimore: Williams & Wilkins, 1989b.

Wu WC, and Pearlman RA: Consent in medical decision-making: The role of communication. Journal of General Internal Medicine, *3*:9-14, 1988.

EPILOGUE

Practice and Self-Awareness

The following will help you analyze how you respond to patients and how you might apply the various communication skills and techniques discussed in this book. Several cases are presented which simulate communication problems found in pharmacy practice. In the first few cases, specific communication skills and strategies are discussed in detail. These comments may help the reader as they consider the remaining situations. The cases are followed by study questions from each of the chapters of the book.

CASE #1

One of your patients, Mrs. Conrad, brings in a new prescription for Dilantin Infatabs®. You know her four-year-old son, Jim, has had several seizures and has had neurological testing.

Pharmacist: Mrs. Conrad, the prescription for Jim is ready. Before you go, I'd like to spend about five minutes discussing this medicine with you. I want to make sure that Jim doesn't run into any problems when he starts taking the medication.

Mrs. Conrad: Fine. I have time now.

Pharmacist: Let's sit over here where we will have some privacy.

Mrs. Conrad: All right.

Pharmacist: Mrs. Conrad, your doctor has prescribed Dilantin® to treat Jim's epilepsy.

Mrs. Conrad: How did you know he has epilepsy?

Pharmacist: Well ... that is the most typical diagnosis for the use of this drug.

Mrs. Conrad: I see.

Pharmacist: Jim is supposed to take the Dilantin® three times a day. You should space the doses as evenly as possible over a 24-hour period. This will mean that you will be giving the Dilantin every eight hours.

Mrs. Conrad: I *know* all that. My doctor went over these instructions quite thoroughly.

Pharmacist: Did he discuss the side effects Jim might have when he begins taking the medicine?

Mrs. Conrad: Yes. He did that quite thoroughly as well.

Pharmacist: Very good. One other thing I am concerned about is establishing a time for taking the medicines that fits into your daily routine. Otherwise it is very difficult to remember to take the medicine. Let's start with the morning — what time does Jim get up?

Mrs. Conrad: Usually around 6:00.

Pharmacist: What time does he go to bed?

Mrs. Conrad: About 9:00.

Pharmacist: If you gave doses at 6:00 in the morning, at 1:30 in the afternoon and at 9:00 at night, that would be close enough to every eight hours. Is there anything you do at 1:30 every day that would help you remember to give Jim his medicine — eat lunch, put him down for a nap, that sort of thing?

Mrs. Conrad: No. We eat lunch at 11:30 and Jim rarely takes a nap anymore.

Pharmacist: You're wearing a digital watch … does it have an alarm you can set?

Mrs. Conrad: Yes, it does.

Pharmacist: I recommend setting it to go off when Jim's afternoon dose of medication is due. Otherwise, setting an alarm at your house or posting a note you will be sure to see at 1:30 will help you remember to give Jim that dose. If you don't do something like this, it is very hard to remember to take a medication when you first start using it.

Mrs. Conrad: The watch alarm is a good suggestion. I'm not good at remembering to give him medicine.

Pharmacist: I am giving you a leaflet that tells more about the medicine, including what to do if you forget to give a dose. Please read it carefully and call me if you have any questions or concerns.

Mrs. Conrad: Thank you.

Pharmacist: Are there any questions you have now or issues you would like to discuss?

Mrs. Conrad: I sure hope this medication works. The seizures were awful to see.

Pharmacist: That must have been very frightening for you.

Mrs. Conrad: It was. I was so scared and felt so helpless.

Pharmacist: It has to be hard to learn to cope with such a disease.

Mrs. Conrad: At least now I know what the problem is and how to handle a seizure when it happens.

Pharmacist: This medication helps a lot of people with epilepsy lead normal lives. We'll work with you to get Jim's dosing plan to be just right for him. And please call me if you have any concerns about his treatment once you get home and start giving Jim the medication.

Mrs. Conrad: Thank you.

Take a minute to analyze the above dialogue in terms of the skills and barriers to effective communication discussed earlier in the text. Examine each of the pharmacist's responses and analyze its effect on the communication process. What pharmacist responses were ineffective and why? How did the patient respond to the pharmacist in these instances? What specifically should the pharmacist have done to improve the communication? What were the positive aspects of the pharmacist's communication? What effective communication skills were utilized? How did these responses seem to affect the patient and the communication process? What assertiveness, empathy, interviewing, assessment, and patient education issues are evident in this exchange? What ethical issues are involved? How well did the pharmacist meet her ethical responsibilities to the patient? What assumptions did she seem to make that may not have been true?

Let's examine the specific pharmacist responses. When she begins the conversation with Mrs. Conrad, she calls her by name, tells her that she wishes to discuss the new prescription and why, tells her how long the consultation will take and gets her consent to proceed. The pharmacist is assertive in initiating communication and shows respect for Mrs. Conrad by explaining the purpose of the consultation and getting her cooperation. She also makes sure they have the privacy necessary to facilitate effective communication. These are all positive responses on the part of the pharmacist.

Problems first appear when the pharmacist starts providing information about the new medication. Her assumption that the physician has diagnosed epilepsy seems presumptuous to the patient's mother and she reacts negatively. This problem could have been avoided if the pharmacist had let the mother tell *her* what the physician had told the mother about the diagnosis and about the new drug treatment. This would have prevented the pharmacist from repeating information about the dosing schedule the mother already knew, which led to impatience on her part. It also would have led to a more thorough assessment of how well informed the mother was about side effects and precautions to follow after Jim begins taking the medication. The closed question "Did [your physician] discuss the side effects Jim might have?" led to a "yes" response, which is inadequate as a way of assessing adequacy of understanding. Without verifying that such understanding exists, the pharmacist cannot assure that informed consent to treatment has taken place.

The pharmacist does a very good job of tailoring the regimen schedule to the patient's daily routine and in suggesting cues or reminders to help the mother remember doses. Such an effort will go a long way in assisting Mrs. Conrad in carrying out the regimen demands. Success in adhering to treatment demands early on leads to increased feelings of self-efficacy or confidence in ability to follow treatment recommendations on the part of patients or patients' care givers.

Finally, the pharmacist showed a great deal of understanding for the difficulties the child's epilepsy presented for the mother. She asked an open-ended question on whether Mrs. Conrad had issues she wished to discuss and was empathic toward her when she expressed her fears and feelings of helplessness. She made it clear that she wanted to work with the mother in establishing effective treatment for her son and that she was available to the mother to discuss concerns she might have in the future.

CASE # 2

You are a new pharmacist practicing in a community pharmacy setting. A patient, Jane Kramer, comes into the pharmacy to get a new prescription for DiaBeta filled. In checking her patient profile, you learn that she is a long-time patron of the pharmacy, is 55 years old, is 5'4" tall and weighs 185 lbs. She has a refill history for Capoten that indicates a pattern of late refills — in fact, the last refill should have run out two weeks ago. She got a new prescription for Clinoril filled three weeks ago and one for erythromycin two weeks ago. The Capoten, Clinoril, and DiaBeta are prescribed by Dr. Sharp and the erythromycin by Dr. Long.

Before you let Ms. Kramer leave the pharmacy with her new prescription, you get her consent to talk with you for approximately ten minutes. What information is it necessary to obtain from Jane Kramer in order to provide a high level of pharmaceutical care? What would you want to know about her and her medication therapy? Phrase questions that you would actually ask her to try to obtain this information. What understanding about Ms. Kramer would you like to have before she leaves your pharmacy? What understanding would you like Ms. Kramer to have before she leaves?

Below are pieces of information about Ms. Kramer that could be obtained in an interview. Which pieces of information about Ms. Kramer were you likely to have obtained by the questions you asked her? What important information would you have likely missed? What assumptions did you make about Ms. Kramer that were not true? What barriers do you think might keep you from getting a complete picture of a patient and her medication therapy?

1. Information should be obtained on all prescription and significant nonprescription medications the patient is currently taking in order to assure that profiles are complete.

    If you assumed that your computer profile about Ms. Kramer provided a complete picture of current prescription medication use, you would not have found out about a Prozac prescription the patient has filled in a pharmacy located next door to the psychiatrist she is currently seeing. The Prozac and psychotherapy have been very effective in treating the patient's depression. In addition, while the patient does know that she is not supposed to take aspirin now that she has started taking Clinoril, she does take OTC ibuprofen for headaches (she takes approximately 2 tablets three times a week).

2. Information should be obtained on chronic medications currently being taken. What does the patient understand about these treatments? How does the patient actually take these medications? What problems does she perceive with their use? Have they been associated with side effects she has been experiencing? How effective have they seemed to be?

    If you had automatically assumed that the late refills on Capoten meant that Ms. Kramer was noncompliant with treatment, you would have been mistaken. This patient is married to a man who recently lost his job; money is extremely tight; and her physician, knowing this, gives her samples of Capoten that she uses to supplement the prescriptions when she is not able to afford to get refills on time. The physician has told the patient that her high blood pressure is under good control. The patient thinks the Clinoril is working well in controlling arthritis pain and she takes the doses as prescribed regardless of level of pain symptoms.

3. Patient response to recently prescribed medications to treat acute conditions should be assessed.

    Ms. Kramer went to a walk-in clinic approximately two weeks ago and was diagnosed with an upper respiratory infection. She was given a prescription for erythromycin which she was supposed to take four times a day. After about four or five days of the 10-day course, she started forgetting doses and finally just quit taking the medication altogether. She still has a cough at night but did not mention this to her physician because she was embarrassed to admit that she had seen a different physician.

4. The possible presence of other medical problems that are not being treated or that her physician is unaware of should be assessed.

    In the case of Ms. Kramer, she is being treated for all of the medical problems she currently has except for the lingering cough of which her physician is unaware.

5. An assessment should be made of what the patient understands about her new medication, DiaBeta. What does she know about diabetes and its treatment? About long-term effects of uncontrolled diabetes? About the name of the drug, its purpose, directions for use, possible side effects, and duration of use? What should she do if she forgets a dose? What are the signs and treatment of hypoglycemia? What are some precautions she should follow when taking the drug? What is the patient supposed to do to monitor control of her condition? What had she been doing before this to treat her symptoms or her condition? What problems did she experience with this treatment? What other medical advice is she supposed to follow in treating her diabetes? How confident is she in her ability to follow treatment demands? What beliefs does she have about her disease and treatment? How confident is she in the effectiveness of treatment? What problems does she foresee?

    The patient has been trying to control her diabetes with diet and exercise as her physician recommended, but with little success. She has been well informed about the treatment, but she has misconceptions about the disease and is not optimistic about her ability to control its progression. She is still supposed to follow the diet and exercise plan. She plans to monitor her blood glucose to measure her progress.

6. Concerns or questions the patient might have about her diseases and/or treatments should be assessed.

    Jane Kramer is extremely upset about her diagnosis of diabetes and discouraged because she has been unable to control it through diet and exercise. Her father had juvenile onset diabetes and died when she was ten of renal failure caused by uncontrolled diabetes. Although the physician did tell her that she had a different type of diabetes, her anxiety and an incomplete explanation on the part of the physician caused her to fail to understand the difference between Type I and Type II diabetes. As a result, the diagnosis is very frightening for her and she lacks confidence in her ability to manage her disease.

CASE #3

Patricia Evans is a community pharmacist. A woman she has never seen before approaches the prescription counter with a prescription for Alupent for a pediatric patient, "John Moore." Analyze the following communication between Patricia Evans and the patient's mother, Ms. Moore.

Pharmacist: Hello. I'm Patricia Evans, the pharmacist here.

Ms. Moore: Hi. I'm Cindy Moore. The prescription is for my son, Johnny.

Pharmacist: Is this the first time you have been to our pharmacy?

Ms. Moore: Yes.

Pharmacist: With people who are coming to our pharmacy for the first time, we like to find out about medications they are currently taking so we can prevent any problems occurring with new medications. If you have about 10 minutes, I'd like to talk with you about the medications Johnny takes. While we're talking, the technician will begin filling your prescription.

Ms. Moore: OK.

Pharmacist: First, how old is Johnny?

Ms. Moore: He's five.

Pharmacist: What medical problems does Johnny have?

Ms. Moore: He has asthma. It's really awful. I get so scared when he has an asthma attack.

Pharmacist: I'm sure with this new medication, we'll be able to prevent those attacks.

Ms. Moore: Yeah. I've heard that before. "Things will get better." Well, things *aren't* getting better.

Pharmacist: I'm sure your doctor is doing all he can.

Ms. Moore: I'm *sure* he is.

Pharmacist: What prescription medications is Johnny currently taking for his asthma?

Ms. Moore: He is taking Somophyllin and will be taking the new prescription I just gave you.

Pharmacist: Do you give the Somophyllin as prescribed?

Ms. Moore: Of course I do!

Pharmacist: How well does Johnny take his medicine?

Ms. Moore: He doesn't like to take it. He spits it out.

Pharmacist: You're going to have to get him to take it better than that. Otherwise, you can't be sure he's getting the full dose.

Ms. Moore: I bet *you* don't have kids.

Pharmacist: What other medication does Johnny take?

Ms. Moore: None.

Pharmacist: Is Johnny allergic to any medication?

Ms. Moore: Yes. He had a reaction to penicillin when he was a baby.

Pharmacist: What happened when he had the reaction?

Ms. Moore: He got a rash and ran a fever.

Pharmacist: Any other allergies to medications?

Ms. Moore: No.

Pharmacist: Let me see if I have everything you've told me — Johnny is taking Somophyllin to treat asthma but has still been having asthma symptoms. He does not like to take the Somophyllin. He is allergic to penicillin. Is there anything else you can think of — other medications he takes or problems he has had with medications?

Ms. Moore: No.

Pharmacist: Now let's discuss the new medication that you will be giving Johnny....

Once again, analyze the above communication in terms of positive and negative aspects of the pharmacist's communication. Examine each pharmacist response and Ms. Moore's reaction to the pharmacist's communication. How could questions have been rephrased to be more effective? What questions should have been asked but were not? What could the pharmacist have said to show more understanding and empathy? What possible drug-related problems were uncovered during the interview? What interventions might the pharmacist initiate to help resolve these drug-related problems?

CASE #4

You are a new pharmacist at a community pharmacy. Eleanor Norton is an 80-year-old woman who comes into your pharmacy and presents complaints of insomnia and mild depression. A look at her computer profile reveals prescriptions for Premarin .625 mg 1 QD and Provera 2.5 mg 1 QD first filled in your pharmacy approximately 1.5 years ago. In addition, she has refill records for Trazodone 50 mg 1 QHS and Xanax .25 mg 1 TID initiated approximately one year ago. Refill records are consistent and do not indicate either late or early refills. Complete demographic and allergy information are on the profile, as are notes that indicate the patient does not smoke and does not consume either caffeine or alcohol.

What further information would you want from Ms. Norton to assess her complaints of insomnia and depression? Phrase the exact questions you would ask her to try to obtain this information.

Now analyze the following exchange between a pharmacist and Ms. Norton in which she attempts to assess her complaints.

Pharmacist: Ms. Norton, I am concerned about your reports of problems sleeping and feelings of depression. I'd like to take about 10 minutes to talk with you about these problems and about the medications you take. This will help me determine things we might do to resolve these problems. Do you have the time now to talk with me?

Patient: Yes, I do.

Pharmacist: Good. Let's sit over here where we have more privacy..... Now, first tell me when you started experiencing the problems sleeping.

Patient: About a year ago. I had problems sleeping and felt moody and tired all the time. This is just not like me. I've always been upbeat and very active. Never had a bit of trouble sleeping.

Pharmacist: Was there anything that happened at that time that might have caused the problem?

Patient: Nothing. I've been widowed for 20 years and have gotten used to living alone. My children live nearby and visit nearly every day. Nothing was any different.

Pharmacist: It must have been frustrating to suddenly feel depressed for no reason you could identify.

Patient: It was. I'm not one to sit around and feel sorry for myself all the time.

Pharmacist: What did you do about the problem at that time?

Patient: I told my doctor and she started giving me the Trazodone and Xanax to try to get me over it.

Pharmacist: And how did that work?

Patient: I think it did help at first. For several months I seemed to feel better. But then the sleep problems started in again. I am very faithful about taking my medicines but they still didn't seem to do the trick. I told my doctor about it but she didn't change my medicines. I read in *Consumer Reports* about the dangers of Xanax in older people, but she seemed to think I should stick with it a while longer.

Pharmacist: How do you take the Trazodone?

Patient: I take it every night at bedtime. Never miss.

Pharmacist: And the Xanax?

Patient: Every eight hours. I set an alarm so I remember them.

Pharmacist: Have you had any problems with the use of either of these medicines?

Patient: Like side effects? Nothing really. The only problem is they don't seem to work.

Pharmacist: That must be discouraging.

Patient: It is. And I'm on a very tight budget. I can't afford to buy medications that aren't doing me any good.

Pharmacist: Let's talk more about the symptoms you currently have. Tell me about the problem sleeping.

Patient: I have trouble getting to sleep every night but that isn't as bad as waking up at 2:00 and not getting back to sleep until 6:00 and waking up again at 8:00. This happens almost every night and has been going on for months. I'm tired all day. I used to garden and belonged to clubs and now I don't want to do anything. I don't even invite friends over for lunch like I used to. I'm just too depressed.

Pharmacist: It sounds like the problems sleeping and the depression have changed your life in profound ways.

Patient: I hate feeling this way. I'm lonely but I know it's because I don't see my friends as much as I used to. I keep hoping the medicines will start working or the doctor will give me something new to take.

Pharmacist: I'll work closely with your doctor to see if we can suggest better treatment for your problems.

Patient: I'd sure appreciate that.

Pharmacist: Now I'd like to find out about other medications you might take. What other prescription medications do you take?

Patient: I take Premarin and Provera, one tablet each every morning. My doctor prescribed it to prevent osteoporosis.

Pharmacist: When did you first begin taking these medications?

Patient: Over a year ago. I never bothered to go to a doctor much and didn't start taking hormones when I was younger like most women do. I didn't need them. I still don't seem to have problems — haven't had any broken bones or other problems which, according to what I have read, go along with osteoporosis.

Pharmacist: Do taking the hormones present any problems for you?

Patient: Not really. I have read that they can cause depression, but when I asked my doctor about it, she told me they were not the cause of my problems.

Pharmacist: I see. Do you take any other prescription medications?

Patient: No. Nothing.

Pharmacist: Now I'd like to discuss medications you take that you can get without a prescription, in a drug store or grocery store.

Patient: I don't like to take anything. I'll take Tylenol if I have a headache, but it has to be pretty bad. I can't remember the last time I've taken anything like that.

Pharmacist: OK. Let me just summarize and you can jump in if I have anything wrong or missed something.... You take Premarin and Provera which you started over a year ago. Approximately one year ago you started experiencing problems with insomnia and depression. Your doctor prescribed Trazodone and Xanax, which seemed to help for several months but then the problems returned. You take no other prescriptions and rarely use nonprescription medications.... Is there anything else you can think of regarding your use of medications?

Patient: No. That's all I can think of.

Pharmacist: Thank you. This information helps me keep track of how you are responding to your treatment. I can then inform you and your physician if I think any problems you are experiencing might be helped by changing your drug therapy. Often, we can't know if a medicine is the best one for you unless we try it and see how it works. I will be communicating with your doctor as soon as I can about your sleep problems and depression and together we'll try to come up with something that is effective in overcoming these problems. I don't want to keep you waiting longer today. I'll call you within the week to discuss our recommendation with you. Will that be OK. with you?

Patient: I'd really appreciate that. Sometimes I'm so flustered when I see my doctor that I don't remember to tell him everything.

Pharmacist: And if you think of anything when you get home, or if you have any concerns about your treatment, please call me. I'll give you my card with my phone number on it. Do you have anything you'd like to discuss right now?

Patient: No. The sleep problem is the main thing I want resolved and we've discussed that pretty thoroughly. I see my doctor in two weeks, so I hope she can do something then to help me.

Critique the pharmacist interview depicted above. What were the strengths and weaknesses of the pharmacist's communication? What further information do you think she should have obtained from the patient? How empathic did she seem?

Now decide which of the points of information obtained in the interview with Ms. Norton you would want to document in the patient's chart. How would you write these notes? What would your purpose be in recording this information?

What drug-related problems or possible drug-related problems were uncovered in the conversation with Ms. Norton? What steps would you now take to try to help the patient resolve these drug-related problems, with the purpose of increasing her quality of life? What action would you take in regard to the prescribing physician? Specify exactly what you would communicate and the method of communication you would choose. What would you do in regard to the patient?

The pharmacist who conducted the interview with Ms. Norton decided to intervene with the prescribing physician. Since the problems Ms. Norton reported had been ongoing and did not seem urgent, the pharmacist decided she could best communicate with the physician in a consult letter. Please critique the letter on the next page. What was the tone the pharmacist was trying to set with the physician? What are the strengths evident in the way the pharmacist approached the communication? What changes would you have made to improve the effectiveness of the written communication?

After critiquing the letter, identify what information contained in the letter and what information from the physician response to the letter you would choose to document in your patient records. How would you record the information? Why would this information be important to you?

In evaluating the consult letter, it is necessary to ask the following questions:

1. Was the correspondence personalized? It should be typed on pharmacy letterhead and personalized to the specific patient rather than having the feel of a "form letter."

2. Was the following information provided?

    a. patient name

    b. date of communication with patient or date of review of patient medication use

PHARMACY LETTERHEAD WITH ADDRESS AND PHONE NUMBER

Jane N. Sellers, M.D.   Current date
1616 N. 50 St.
Cooperstown, NY

Dear Dr. Sellers:

   Yesterday I spoke with one of your patients, Eleanor Norton, who conveyed to me her concerns about problems with insomnia and depression. She reported that the Trazodone and Xanax you prescribed for her condition seemed to work for several months, but then the symptoms returned. The symptoms have led her to severely restrict her activities and contacts with friends, which she reports has had a negative effect on her quality of life. I would like to work with you to devise an alternative treatment for Ms. Norton that might relieve the symptoms she reports. I can assist you in closely monitoring her response to treatment to see if changes we make resolve the problems.

   I believe there are three alternative avenues we might explore to resolve the patient's problems. The focus might be on altering the hormone replacement therapy, on choosing an alternate antidepressant such as fluoxetine, or on altering the benzodiazepine therapy. The onset of depressive symptoms shortly after initiation of hormone replacement therapy suggests the possibility that the hormone therapy is causing the depression. I, therefore, think this should be our first line of attack. I am enclosing a recent article in [*Name of Journal*] which suggests that hormone replacement therapy may not be necessary in women over 75 with no history of bone fractures or other indications of severe osteoporosis. The authors note that most of the loss of bone density occurs prior to age 75. They also review the evidence that a side effect for many patients is depression. The recommendation of these authors is use of calcium and Vitamin D supplements only. While there is certainly variation in medical practice on this issue, I think the decreased quality of life of Ms. Norton due to the depression, which could be tied to the hormone therapy, makes an alternative treatment worth considering. You may feel more confident in making this decision if a bone density evaluation of Ms. Norton was first conducted. My only concern here would be with the cost of the procedure, given the limited income Ms. Norton reports.

   If you decide to discontinue hormone replacement therapy, I plan to call Ms. Norton every two weeks to assess her response to the alteration and will update you on her progress. If she responds well, we could then discuss gradually reducing and eventually eliminating the Trazodone and Xanax. If response is not as we would hope, we could then discuss an alternative approach to address the problem. Ms. Norton informed me that she has an appointment to see you in two weeks. Please keep me informed of any changes that you make in her therapy so that I may be of as much assistance as possible.

   I hope to be able to work with you in helping Ms. Norton. I welcome the opportunity to discuss alternative approaches to resolving Ms. Norton's depression. Please call me at your earliest convenience.

Sincerely,

Paula T. Singer, Pharm.D.
Registered Pharmacist

c. concerns expressed by the patient or uncovered in drug use review

d. identification of any verified or potential drug-related problem (this could include misuse of the medication by the patient, presence of a possible medical problem not currently being treated, or problems related to current medication therapy)

e. clarification of the optimal therapeutic outcome

f. description of appropriate alternative approaches to resolving drug-related problem(s)

g. recommendation as to the preferred alternative and specific recommendations for implementation (e.g., dosing recommendations for selected drugs) which are tailored to the patient's needs

h. suggestion for an appropriate monitoring plan, along with specific actions you will undertake to assist in monitoring patient response

3. Was recommendation supported with citations from current, accepted literature sources?

4. Did the letter welcome a two-way dialogue with the physician?

5. Was the tone one which emphasized helping the patient rather than promoting the pharmacist?

Now, let's consider the information you identified for documentation in the pharmacy patient profile of Ms. Norton. This information should include:

1. Date of conversation with the patient.

2. The concerns expressed by the patient about the ongoing problems of insomnia and depression.

3. Actions initiated and specific recommendations made to either the patient or the physician to resolve the problem.

4. A monitoring plan with specific dates of pharmacist follow-up with both patient and physician in order to assess resolution of the problem and determine further steps that may be needed to optimize therapy.

CASE #5

Bob Hunter is a 40-year-old male who suffers from seasonal allergies. His allergies have become worse since he moved to a state well known for its bothersome plant life. Typically, he can expect his eyes to become watery and red, his nose to run, and his head to ache mildly. On this occasion these symptoms appear along with a sore throat and a more severe headache. He felt he had strep throat and so he sought the services of a physician. The physician assured him the symptoms were his allergies "kicking up" and that the sore throat and headache were due to sinus drainage. The physician gave Bob the following prescription, which he brought to his pharmacist:

Bob Hunter
Rx: Decon-Histamine Tab
#60
Sig: i am, i pm,
J. Smith MD

What should the pharmacist verify before and after filling this prescription? What questioning could the pharmacist do to keep the counseling encounter to less than a minute and still fulfill her OBRA obligations?

HINTS: By using a few simple open-ended questions, as described in Chapters 7 and 8, the pharmacist could verify that the medication is being taken for seasonal allergies, even though the patient's physical appearance probably suggests it. Also verification that these symptoms are not the side effects of any other OTC or Rx medication is needed. Finally through open-ended questions the pharmacist should verify that the patient understands the directions for use and any anticipated side effects such as drowsiness.

CASE #6

Elderly men and women are special opportunities for pharmacists as they account for 30% of all Rx medication taken in the USA and 40% of all OTC medication. As a group, two out of three elderly take at least one medication daily. The sheer volume of medications taken by the elderly, plus their well-known risk factors (i.e., cognitive problems, polypharmacy, living alone, economic issues, multiple medical problems affecting altered physiology, and loss of sight, hearing, taste, and smell, as well as, jobs, friends and family) lead to high incidences of medication misadventures. Keeping these issues in mind, respond to the following encounter:

> Nellie Cistis, age 83, has been a member of a large managed-care plan since its inception in 1975. She became a member when part of her husband's employee benefits package when his employer converted shortly after his retirement. She has always had her prescriptions filled at the clinic pharmacy run by the HMO. On this occasion she enters the pharmacy to pick up refills for two of her medications, a diuretic and a digitalis glycoside. Nellie is greeted by the pharmacist:

Pharmacist: Hello Nellie! I bet you are having a good day today.

Nellie: Not really, but why are you so sure?

Pharmacist: Because with all this rain we've been having it's gotta be good for the crops and making the grass green.

Nellie: Well I guess so.

Pharmacist: Here are your medicines. Let's see, you take one of each once a day, except the little white one is every other day. Right?

Nellie: Yup, I think you've got it.

Pharmacist: You have been on this stuff a long time, haven't you?

Nellie: Yup, 'bout a decade.

Pharmacist: You're not having any problems with them, are you?

Nellie: Well, I mustn't be, I'm still around ain't I? Say, why all the questions?

Pharmacist: It's our new policy to talk to people. There is a new law that says we need to talk more to customers.

Nellie: It's about time!

Pharmacist: Well Nellie, y'all have a good one.

How could the pharmacist have prepared this elderly patient for a counseling encounter? How could the pharmacist establish a more respectful relationship? How could the pharmacist assess and respond to any of Nellie's needs related to sight, hearing, or memory loss? Could the pharmacist have helped Nellie identify events in her daily living habits to help remind her to take her medication consistently? What simple sentences could the pharmacist have used to assure Nellie's understanding of how and why she takes her medicines? Rewrite the pharmacist's leading, restrictive, and judgmental dialogue in order to let Nellie respond with items that are important to her.

CASE #7

Since the incidence of HIV infection is rising worldwide, particularly in heterosexual women, adolescents, and IV drug users, pharmacists, like any other health professional, have a responsibility to be well educated regarding this disease. Respond to the following scenario:

Mary Jane Marvel is a 29-year-old woman attending a prestigious state university. She is pretty and the life of a lot of parties. For the past semester, she has had a nagging vaginal infection. Her sorority volunteered to conduct a blood drive for the local Red Cross Chapter and, like every other sorority sister, Mary Jane tried to give blood. However, she tested positive for HIV and was refused. She became scared and angry and went to a doctor, where she was still too confused to talk about the HIV test but did talk about the nagging vaginal infection. The doctor gave her a prescription for a common antifungal/yeast infection. She now takes it to the campus pharmacy. She stands off to one side while the pharmacist fills the prescription. The pharmacist notices her behavior and leaves the prescription counter to talk with her.

Pharmacist: Hello Miss Marvel. I am Francine Friendly, and the pharmacist who filled your prescription. May I talk to you a little bit about it?

Mary Jane: Sure, why not? (said nervously)

Pharmacist: Well, I was watching you a moment ago and you seem full of emotion. I cannot tell if you are scared, angry, or embarrassed. Would you like to tell me a little bit about how you are felling?

Mary Jane: How would you feel if you had to stick that stuff inside you?

Pharmacist: I can tell you are more than embarrassed — you are angry over something. Is there anything else besides this infection that has you anxious and worried?

Mary Jane: Well its pretty darn personal. Why should I confide in you?

Pharmacist: For a lot of reasons, but chief among them is the fact that I am always here to listen. I am a knowledgeable health professional, but most of all I truly do care.

Mary Jane: Well, I guess I must tell someone before I bust.

Pharmacist: I do respect your trust and confidence, but before we talk, let's step over here to a little more quiet area that will assure us privacy.

Mary Jane: Well, I failed an HIV test and I am scared that I am gonna die.

Analyze the pharmacist's ability to take Mary Jane into /her confidence. Discuss the barriers a pharmacist may have to an HIV patient, beyond the typical ones of lacking in self-confidence, reluctance to take time, failure to recognize patient needs, and just plain poor communication skills. In other words, discuss this pharmacist's ability to convey that she is ready to listen, and is believable, likable, and trustworthy! Discuss the following guidelines that help one become an active listener:

Do you listen to understand?
Do you empathize to show you care?
Do you hold back arguments so as not to appear judgmental?
Do you ask questions to clarify?
Do you repeat or summarize to verify?

Every pharmacist is aware that HIV infection leads to devastating illness and that it does not discriminate by age, race, sex, sexual preference, or social class. Discuss how education is a great hope that can lead to changes in behavior that reduce transmission of HIV. Discuss the pharmacist's role in educating patients so that she may have a significant impact on the optimal outcomes of medication used by HIV patients.

CASE #8

Mrs. Hope is 70 and she takes care of her husband, John, who is the same age. John is confined to home because of his Alzheimer's condition. Mrs. Hope has taken John to a physician for a checkup and now visits the outpatient clinic pharmacy in the hospital where the physician holds privileges.

Pharmacist: Good morning, Mrs. Hope. How are you today?

Mrs. Hope: I'm OK, but I'm concerned about these new prescriptions. One is for me, the other is for my husband, John.

Pharmacist: May I please read them?

Mrs. Hope: Yes, go ahead.

Pharmacist: Which one concerns you?

Mrs. Hope: They both do. The one for John — I was never told why it was prescribed. The second one for me is something I've never had before.

Pharmacist: Well, John's prescription is for a diuretic. That means it's a water pill and it works to remove extra fluid from inside the body. Your prescription is what we call a nonsteroidal inflammatory drug. It's used to reduce the inflammation and pain associated with conditions like arthritis.

Mrs. Hope: But John has Alzheimer's and I do not have arthritis. The doctor is new and only saw us once. Why would he prescribe such stuff?

Can you put yourself into Mrs. Hope's place? What could she be feeling? What could her needs be other than the need for information? What open-ended questions could the pharmacist have used to initiated the conversation and prevent making false assumptions? What false assumptions contributed to the pharmacists ineffectiveness?

Mrs. Hope is obviously the care giver and, as such, communication with her requires special strategies. After making sure the drugs prescribed are appropriate, what could the pharmacist have done to assure that both patients understand their medication regimens? What could the pharmacist have done or said to encourage and support Mrs. Hope in the care of her husband?

CASE #9

This situation takes place in the small rural town of Taylor, Georgia. Taylor is the home of the county hospital. About ten physicians and two pharmacies (one chain store and one independent) provide health services to the town's inhabitants. Taylor has a racial mix of about 50% White, 40% Black, and 10% Hispanic.

The case involves Mrs. Ernestine Johnson and her son David. David is a six-year-old Black child who tested positive for HIV two years ago. Six months ago he showed slight symptoms of Pneumocystis carinii pneumonia. Since that time he has been given Bactrim suspension prophylaxically (one teaspoonful daily). The Johnsons moved to Taylor because David was not allowed to go to school in Jackson, Georgia, where they had lived for 15 years.

Mrs. Johnson and David enter Fred Schneider's pharmacy for the first time to obtain a new supply of Bactrim and also some Tylenol with Codeine elixir. Betty, the pharmacist, recognizes Mrs. Johnson and David from a picture which appeared in the town's weekly newspaper. An article discussed the arrival of the "AIDS child" at the county grammar school. Many of the town's residents, including Betty, were not too excited about David's being allowed to attend school with their children.

Mrs. Johnson approaches the prescription counter with the two prescriptions and greets Betty, the pharmacist, with a warm smile. Betty kind of grunts "Good morning" as she takes the prescriptions. The following conversation transpires:

Betty: What are these for?

Mrs. Johnson: Something for his lungs. One of them helps with the pain.

Betty: He's got AIDS doesn't he? This may help him for a while, but it's not going to cure him.

Betty retreats behind the prescription counter and gives the prescriptions to her assistant so that the labels can be typed while she prepares the drugs.

Assistant: Mrs. Johnson, who's this doctor? I can't read his handwriting.

Mrs. Johnson: That would be Dr. Dennis. He was seeing David in Morgantown where we used to live.

Betty (to the assistant): Can't fill these, they might be forgeries. They should come from a local doctor, but I don't know who will treat an AIDS patient, especially the son of a drug addict.

Betty: Mrs. Johnson, I'm sorry. You'll have to get these written by a local physician. I could recommend Dr. Wright, he sees most of the Medicaid patients in Taylor. His office is next to the county hospital.

Mrs. Johnson: I thought I could get these filled anywhere. I'd rather not run around all over town with David.

Betty: Sorry, rules are rules. We close tonight at 9:00 sharp. Bye.

Mrs. Johnson and David exit.

What would you call the mental image the pharmacist had about the patient? Do you think stereotypes influence a pharmacist's behavior?

The authors recognize Betty's behavior, and the attitude manifested, are unacceptable. this is not professional demeanor. If allowed, these traits can destroy the professional's ability to establish a helpful relationship with the patient-customer. It is helpful to recognize any evidence of such attitudes and make certain they do not appear in oneself or staff. What should the owner of this pharmacy say to Betty once the conversation had been overheard? What other communication problems did you see?

CASE #10

An elderly patient on a fixed income enters a pharmacy to discuss the following problem:

Patient: Last week I had my Inderal prescription refilled and you shorted me five tablets. Instead of 90 tablets, you only gave me 85. You tried to cheat me! This is not the first time, either. It has happened before and I am really upset.

How would you response to this individual? What communication techniques could you use to resolve this issue?

CASE #11

A women enters the pharmacy to discuss the following situation:

Patient: I recently found a prescription for Penicillin for my boyfriend from the county's STD (sexually transmitted diseases) clinic. This prescription was filled at this pharmacy three days ago and I want to know what it is used for. What's going on here?

What would you say to this patient? What important communication and ethical issues are involved?

CASE #12

A patient who looks somewhat depressed approaches the prescription counter.

Patient: Boy, I can't believe what is happening to me. I went to the doctor because I was feeling kind of low. She gave me a prescription for

Dalmane 30 mg. It certainly helps me sleep, but I still feel depressed. Did you ever wonder if life was worth the hassle?

How would you respond to this person? What is your role in this situation?

CASE #13

A patient, Ms. Reynolds, enters a pharmacy, having just come from her physician's office.

Ms. Reynolds: My doctor just gave me a prescription for Methotrexate and did not tell me anything about it! What's it used for?

Pharmacist: Gee whiz, I am kind of busy right now to talk, but it can be used to treat cancer.

Ms. Reynolds (frantic and angry): What?! Oh my goodness! I can't believe I have cancer. I can't believe this. Am I going to die? I'm not going to take this stuff — it will probably make me sicker. I'm out of here.

How could the pharmacist have handled this situation differently? What would you have said to the patient? Would you call anyone else about this? If so, whom?

CASE #14

A husband comes into your pharmacy to discuss a problem his wife has been having lately.

Husband: My wife has been taking a tranquilizer, diazepam I believe, for about four months after she pinched a nerve in the back of her neck at work. She has been acting different lately and I am afraid she is becoming addicted to this drug. She is also drinking more than she used to. She seems to be very moody — anxious one moment and quiet the next. I went through her things and found several prescription bottles from different physicians and from other pharmacies. What should I do? Is there any hope?

What would you say to this husband? What is your role in this interaction? Would you call anyone else about this? If so, whom?

CASE 15

You are a pharmacist in a pharmacy located in a medical building, and a woman, Cynthia Jackson, whom you recognize but do not know, enters your pharmacy. Cynthia is a 22-year-old college student and has little money to pay for medication. She has chronic sinusitis and finally realized she needed to see an ear, nose, and throat specialist. Cynthia visited Dr. Sampson. who practices in your building. You know Dr. Sampson to be a good physician, but one who lacks interpersonal skills at times. She prescribed a new third-generation cephalosporin product that costs $75. After you dispense the prescription, counsel Cynthia about the medication, and tell her the price, Cynthia states, "That darn Dr. Sampson didn't help me very much. All she wanted to talk about is my acne! And how do you get off charging me so much for that stupid antibiotic?"

What feelings do you sense coming from Cynthia? How would you respond to Cynthia? What kind of recommendations would you give her?

CASE 16

It is your first day back to work after a vacation. While you were gone, a substitute pharmacist who was not familiar with your pharmacy worked for you. A patient, Sandy Franklin, enters the pharmacy and tries to get your attention. Sandy has been coming to your pharmacy for some time for an antihistamine for her allergies. She states, "Hey, I think you screwed up. These antihistamine tablets say Tylenol #3 on them. It's a good thing I didn't take any as it looks like someone gave me the wrong drug. What's going on?"

What would you say to Sandy? What special communication skills might you use? What would you say to the relief pharmacist?

CASE 17

A muscular college student appears at your pharmacy asking many questions about anabolic steroid use and its side effects. The student claims the information is for a paper that he is writing for his sports medicine class. As you continue the conversation, you get the feeling that this young man is using the steroids himself and has been frightened by a current article published in local press.

What would you say to this student? What type of communication skills might you use?

CASE 18

Jackie, a neighbor of yours, just stopped into your pharmacy to ask you for five Tylenol #3 tablets. Her prescription has run out and she has not had time to call her physician until today. She states that when she called the office for a refill, the nurse told her that her doctor was out of town for the weekend and that she would have to see another physician for a refill. The original prescription was not filled at your pharmacy. In fact, Jackie is not sure which pharmacy filled it first. Jackie states, "Boy, I'm really in a bind. My head hurts and I really need these pills. You've really got to help me out with this one."

How would you handle this situation? What would you say to her? What if she really persists and promises to see the doctor first thing Monday morning?

CASE 19

You are a pharmacist working in a community pharmacy. Mrs. Elliott enters the prescription area to pick up a medication. Mrs. Elliott is a relatively new patient to your pharmacy and has been taking medication for high blood pressure for about four years.

1. You hand her the prescription and say, "I notice that it has been a while since you last got this medication refilled." In

communicating with Mrs. Elliott, which aspect of communication contributes the most in the transmission of your message to her?

a. Level of empathy
b. Tone of voice
c. Nonverbal aspects
d. Amount of privacy
e. b and c

2. Mrs. Elliott seems to be reluctant to answer your direct questions about her compliance with her high blood pressure medication. What type of questions should you ask to draw her out?

a. Open-ended
b. Closed-ended
c. Leading
d. None of the above

3. Mrs. Elliott's reluctance to speak with you may be due to her perception of you as a pharmacist. Which of the following could result in distortions in interpersonal perception?

a. Conflicting values
b. Stereotyping
c. Personal concerns
d. All of the above
e. None of the above

4. Mrs. Elliott states, "I'm tired of taking this medication. Sometimes I don't take them like I should." You respond by saying, "How long have you been taking this medication, Mrs. Elliott? Is it causing you any particular side effects?" Your response is an example of what type of response?

a. Advising
b. Quizzing
c. Analyzing
d. Evaluating
e. Focusing

5. You go on to say, "Now, Mrs. Elliott, you shouldn't worry too much about that. It happens to a lot of people. Everything will work out if you take your medications correctly." This is an example of what type of response?

   a. Advising
   b. Reassuring
   c. Warning
   d. Judging
   e. Understanding

Answers to questions 1 through 5: e, a, d, b, b.

STUDY QUESTIONS

Prologue

1. Describe the societal need for "pharmaceutical care."

2. Recall the two primary functions of communication between health professionals and patients.

3. Describe critical points in the communication process between patient and professional when outcomes can be affected.

Chapter 1

1. There are five components in the communications model. Can you describe them?

2. Where do the meanings of messages come from?

3. What happens when verbal and nonverbal messages are not congruent?

4. How can misperceptions be minimized?

5. What role do self- and process-awareness play?

Chapter 2

1. How do perceptions interfere with communications?

2. What is meant by "Our perception of a message is affected by our perception of the individual."

3. What are two ways you can prevent misunderstandings?

4. Why is it important to ask for feedback?

5. How do stereotypes influence perception?

6. What constitutes the perception of credibility?

Chapter 3

1. How much of communication is attributed to its nonverbal component? Why is this so?

2. What is the importance of cue clusters?

3. Of all the ways we communicate nonverbally, which is the most facilitative?

4. List the many ways that body language can improve your role as a pharmacist.

5. Differentiate between "kinesics" and "proxemics."

6. Examine your own nonverbal behavior and list ways you may overcome any distracting styles.

Chapter 4

1. Explain to someone the meaning of "The number of potential barriers is so great, it's a wonder any communication takes place at all."

2. Argue for and against pharmacists' dispensing from a raised platform.

3.   What is the first step in removing environmental and personal barriers to communication?

4.   What are at least three patient barriers that inhibit communication?

5.   How can the inherent nature of pharmacy practice inhibit good communication?

Chapter 5

1.   Describe the four skills of effective listening; i.e., summarizing, paraphrasing, empathic responding, and nonverbal attending.

2.   Empathic responding has several positive effects. What are they?

3.   Discuss how active listening can be inhibited by stereotyping, depersonalizing, and controlling.

Chapter 6

1.   Compare assertiveness to passivity and aggressiveness.

2.   In what way(s) should pharmacists be assertive with patients? With physicians? With colleagues?

3.   Describe a way to handle criticism without losing self-esteem or mutual respect.

4.   How can assertiveness be used to resolve conflict?.

5.   What is "fogging?"

Chapter 7

1.   What are the critical components of an effective interview?

2.   Why are people better senders of messages than receivers?

3. What are the differences between open-ended and closed-ended questions, and when should each be used?

4. What are five techniques that improve telephone productivity?

5. Would you agree that good interviewing is a learned process? Why?

Chapter 8

1. What is most likely a reason for a pharmacist's inability to help patients take medication as prescribed?

2. What false assumptions do pharmacists often make that cloud otherwise clear communication?

3. What are several techniques that assist a pharmacist in assessing a patient's knowledge about medication?

4. Can you describe at least five techniques that help you "partner" with patients to motivate them into compliance with therapy?

5. Describe several special communication techniques that can be used to effectively improve a pharmacist-patient encounter.

Chapter 9

1. What impact does aging have on learning, memory, and recall?

2. Is there such a thing as a generation gap when counseling patients? If so, explain.

3. What is aphasia, and how can you communicate with a patient who has it?

4. Describe your feelings about the terminally ill and how you could best communicate with them.

5.   What are some of the special communication problems that arise from interactions with care givers?

Chapter 10

1.   Describe "beneficence" and compare it to "fidelity."

2.   State some of the limitations of "informed consent."

3.   Describe the six stages of moral reasoning and list why people do not reach them all.

4.   Describe a rationale for pharmacists to use when resolving ethical dilemmas.

TABLE 1

Eleven Facets That Influence How You C.O.M.M.U.N.I.C.A.T.E. With Patients

C	Communication is a learned skill; your effectiveness is based upon personal choices, attitudes, and beliefs.
O	Openness and trust will develop when active listening and effective feedback are used.
M	Messages mean more when there is congruence between the words and the patient's underlying feelings.
M	Make an effort to listen to yourself. Recall how you respond to situations and see if you recognize any patterns.
U	Use energy and time effectively when you believe you can help; otherwise, do not waste time and energy when you assess that you can do nothing.
N	Nervousness when communicating can best be minimized by developing a positive self-image.
I	Injury to effective communication will occur when you dominate the interaction with technical jargon and unfamiliar words.
C	Communication is a fragile process; if you change it only slightly, you can distort its meaning.
A	Avoid communicating ambiguous nonverbal cues through your facial expressions and body language.
T	Touching, listening, and a kind word are three ways to remove communication barriers.
E	Effective communication requires you to verify the meanings in a message and to accept in a nonjudgmental way the feelings and rights of others.

	TABLE 2
	Ten Techniques That Will Grow Your C.O.U.N.S.E.L.I.N.G. Skills
C	Conduct your counseling in a quiet, designated area to reduce patient anxiety.
O	Open the counseling dialogue by introducing yourself. Speak slowly, maintain eye contact, and avoid professional jargon or multisyllable words.
U	Use mild statements instead of strong ones, which are more threatening.
N	Never disagree with a patient. Instead, offer optional ideas or viewpoints for consideration.
S	Save calling a patient by first name until he gives you permission to do so.
E	Express yourself to show that you tailor each situation to fit each patient.
L	Look like a professional in dress and deportment.
I	Investigate different listening/responding patterns.
N	Never forget that illness or an unfamiliar situation may impair the patient's ability to accept counseling.
G	Get directly to the point by explaining exactly what will take place.

	TABLE 3
	Ten Tips and Tactics That Will Help Improve Patient Compliance
C	Correct misconceptions by identifying the patient's understanding, attitudes, beliefs, and experience about the condition and medication.
O	Open the package or vial to show the patient the actual product.
M	Make time for the patient to be included in any decision making regarding the medication regimens, especially if the decision is to revolve around life events.
P	Provide reinforcement and positive rewards for compliant behavior. Consider patient contracts.
L	Leave written patient information leaflets (PILs) only as an adjunct to and not as a substitute for face-to-face dialogue.
I	Inform the patient of the risks of noncompliance as well as of measurable expected outcomes.
A	Assure the patient that you share in the treatment goals, that the patient's confidentiality is respected, and that you may collaborate with other care givers or providers, especially if there will be a need to change therapy to avoid side effects.
N	Never assume the patient can remain compliant alone; when appropriate, suggest that family, friends, and others become involved.
C	Congratulate the patient for being compliant, especially if he has been able to self-monitor therapy.
E	Evaluate compliance behavior by contacting patients who miss refills.

Index

Page numbers in *italics* denote figures; page numbers followed by t indicate tables.